"Asmaa Hussein. opening. This book is the journey of a courageous woman, a committed wife and a sincere and principled believer. She makes sense of a dramatic experience while remaining faithful to both her values and hopes. Having lost her beloved husband and as she continues to strive for justice and dignity, she is so right in recalling this fundamental truth: 'Nothing is permanent. Not even pain.'"*

Dr. Tariq Ramadan

"Asmaa's heartfelt prose skillfully takes us on a journey of wisdom and insight that could only be forged by experiencing great pain with courage. Her words remind us of just how fragile and short-lived the realities we cling to are, while calling us to look through them to the only permanent truth as our true sanctuary."

Dalia Mogahed

"A Temporary Gift is a moving tour de force that leaves the reader emotionally drained, yet spiritually recharged. Ms. Hussein has succeeded in chronicling the tragic death of her husband at the hands of Egypt's new regime and how that dramatic and unexpected turn of events has caused her to find renewed strength in her faith and family."

Dr. Yasir Qadhi

1

"I am taken aback by what I have read. The emotional, mental, and spiritual roller coaster that I thought only I had gone through in my time in solitary, Asmaa has gone through. I never imagined that anyone outside of prison could have possibly gone through that bumpy ride. Asmaa captures the complexity of feeling hope and desperation simultaneously. A spiritually uplifting read and a story of unshakable trust in the wisdom of God in the face of adversity."

Mohamed Soltan
Egyptian activist and former detainee
at Al-Aqrab prison in Cairo, Egypt

"In my life I haven't read a text so delicate and touching... I read the whole book on my way back from Nigeria where I was visiting my childhood city of Lagos. For the whole journey of seven hours I wept while reading this journal of enlightenment and humanity...

"I didn't meet Brother Amr but for sure he is and will always be in my du'as for shedding light and inspiring me and everyone he knew through his deeds and life. He lived in a way I hope I can live, and died raising his voice against the oppressors.

"This is a book of wise thoughts and words. I recommend it for everyone."

Abdullah Elshamy

Al-Jazeera journalist and former detainee
at Al-Aqrab prison in Cairo, Egypt

"This reader cannot help but have profound admiration for the beautiful patience of Asmaa Hussein. Not an easy patience that slips in peacefully as if from a dream, but a biting forbearance through the persistent struggle of anguish and against the hopelessness of loss.

"Asmaa, by way of painfully arresting prose and poetry, tells the story of her husband Amr who, after just two years of marriage, was tragically murdered during a peaceful protest in Alexandria, Egypt. The reader feels a commanding sense of sorrow listening to Asmaa wrestle living with the death of her beloved. Yet, it is much more a breathing story of redemption and the burning renewal of one's faith through tribulation. It is through this tribulation that Asmaa teaches herself, and by virtue the reader, of the immediacy of repairing your relationship with Allah now, before we are ultimately called to the grave."

Dr. Waleed Basyouni

"Asmaa Hussein's story is a story of love, injustice and hope. Her book is a dive in the swirling worlds of feelings and spirituality. Asmaa sees her love being taken away from her in a horrible act of injustice. Gradually, she finds solace in her faith. A beautiful quest for serenity and acceptance."

Dr. Monia Mazigh

3

A Temporary Gift:

Reflections on Love, Loss, and Healing

ASMAA HUSSEIN

A Temporary Gift:
Reflections on Love, Loss, and Healing

Published by:
Ruqaya's Bookshelf
Toronto, Ontario, Canada
www.ruqayasbookshelf.com
ISBN: 978-0-9947501-2-9

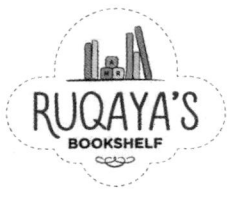

Cover photo by Naoma Khan
Cover design by Islam Farid
Edited by Shoilee Khan
Copy edited by Amina Sadler
Design and typesetting by Calix Ltd

Printed and bound in Canada

In the name of Allah, the Most Beneficent,
the Most Merciful

For Amr's parents, Ragaa and Mohamed: never will Allah (swt) allow the deeds of His servants to go to waste.

For Amr: in the hopes that sharing these memories will cause one person somewhere to make *du'a* for you, to be a better spouse, to have empathy with families who have lost their loved ones, or to make the most out of every moment.

For Ruqaya: that you may know Amr, that you may understand love, that you may aspire to patience.

They say the moon only shines in the darkness of night because it's reflecting the light of the sun...

Isn't it strange that they should be so far from one another, moving along two separate paths that will never meet in this world, and yet their purposes and movements are so intertwined?

Though you have gone and the darkness of night has enveloped us, my heart still reflects what remains of your love and light. It pierces the darkness and illuminates our path so that we may walk forward.

Thank you, my sun.

Amr Kassem 1987-2013

Table of Contents

Note to the Reader

Arabic words and phrases appear in italics in the text. Definitions can be found in the Glossary at the end of the book.

The translations of the meanings of the verses of the Qur'an in this book are taken, with some minor changes, from:

- *The Qur'ân: Arabic Text with Corresponding English Meanings* by Saheeh International.
- *Interpretation of the Meanings of the Noble Qur'ân in the English Language* by Dr. Muhammad Taqi-ud-Deen al-Hilali and Dr. Muhammad Muhsin Khan.
- *The Meaning of the Glorious Qur'an* by Muhammed Marmaduke Pickthall.
- *The Meaning of the Holy Qur'an* by Abdullah Yusuf Ali.

Abbreviations for honorifics used in this book:

(swt): *subhanahu wa ta'ala:* the Exalted; used with the name of Allah.

(saws): *sall-Allahu 'alayhi wa sallam:* may the peace and blessings of Allah be upon him; used with the name of Prophet Muhammad.

(as): *'alayhi salam:* may peace be upon him; used with the names of prophets and messengers.

(ra): *radi Allahu 'anhu:* may Allah be pleased with him; used after the name of a male Companion of the Prophet (saws).

(rah): *radi Allahu 'anha:* may Allah be pleased with her; used after the name of a female Companion of the Prophet (saws).

(rahum): *radi Allahu 'anhum:* may Allah be pleased with them; used when more than one Companion of the Prophet (saws) is mentioned.

Introduction

My Amr.

It was in his heart that my heart found a home after much wandering and loneliness. It was his heart that said to mine: *you will never be frightened or sad while you're with me*. His heart spoke the truth because our life together was full of unmitigated feelings of safety and joy.

Even in the difficult times that every marriage stumbles upon, our hearts were two halves of one. We balanced each other so perfectly that at first it was hard to believe. He was calm when I was angry; I was calm when he was angry. He lifted my sadnesses and I lifted his. One meaningful embrace from him could melt away all my worries. One moment of looking into his eyes, our hands clasped, would calm my nerves and make me believe to my very core that everything would be fine.

My Amr.

He was loved and respected by all who knew him. He could never be in anyone's company without bringing a smile to that person's face. He inspired ease in hearts. He raised people's spirits and hopes. He was unlike anyone I had ever met.

When Allah (swt) places love in your heart for your spouse – the kind of love so deep that it is unaffected by day-to-day stresses; the kind of love that pushes you to be a better, kinder person; the kind of love that makes it seem like you are one soul living in two bodies – it is nothing short of a sign, a miracle, an *ayah*.

In the short period of time between marrying Amr and losing him in one quick moment of violence, I was blessed with his company and an uncomplicated love that not everyone has the privilege of experiencing. Our love was indeed an *ayah*.

{And of His signs is that He created for you from yourselves mates that you may find tranquility in them; and He placed between you affection and mercy. Indeed in that are signs for a people who give thought.}   *(ar-Room 30:21)*

An *ayah* or sign is given to people by Allah in order to direct them, to guide them, and to lead them back to Him.

In both life and death, Amr's example always led me back to Allah.

Some people think love is random, some think it's a simple human instinct to procreate, and some even try to boil it down to the science of chemicals and pheromones. True love, though, whose source is *al-Wadood* – the Most Loving – cannot be touched or seen or measured. How can it be when it is a sign and miracle of Allah?

Allah placed that kind of love between our hearts.

Finding Amr

Before Amr, my life was good. I was blessed with a supportive family and wonderful friends. I had just graduated with a Master of Social Work; to the outside world, everything seemed to be going right for me. However, my heart felt an emptiness that I didn't understand how to fill.

I thought that if I took up a few hobbies and spent time with my friends and family, that void would disappear. Even then, though, my heart was constantly tugging at me as if to say: *You have too much love to give. It needs somewhere to go.*

It was true. I did have an overwhelming amount of love in my heart. It was also true that there was nowhere for it to go. Numerous times, at the behest of family and friends, I met potential spouses. Each time I met someone new, though, there was always something about him that didn't sit well with me. The painfully honest truth was that the more I learned about the characteristics of most men, the more I became disillusioned with the idea of marriage.

I had a conversation with a friend about a month before I met Amr. I told her, "I've reconciled myself to the fact that I may never marry. I have considered a number of men and have been disappointed with them all. Perhaps I am meant to be alone and that's okay. I will live my life as best as I can, I will contribute to my community in the best way that I know how and this will fulfill me. This will be enough for me."

I was exhausted from being disappointed so often. I decided I would just stop trying. My heart needed a break.

A few short weeks later, I met Amr.

Out of frustration I had resigned myself to a life of being alone, but Allah (swt) had something different in mind. He had a gift waiting for me.

One of Allah's names is *al-Wahhab,* which means the Bestower of Gifts. He gives us gifts for different reasons.

He may give a gift solely out of love for His slave. He may see that His slave is distant from Him so He gives her a beautiful gift to bring her back to thanking Him.

For the life of me, I didn't understand why I deserved to be married to someone who was so perfect for me. Just weeks before I'd met Amr, I had totally given up on marriage and no longer wanted to pursue anything related to it. *Al-Wahhab* was adamant about bringing him into my life, however, because He knew Amr was a gift that would cause me to be grateful.

Throughout this period of time, Allah (swt) was showing me that it is not up to me to close a door when He wills it to be open. A few years later, I would learn that it is not up to me to keep a door open that He wishes to be closed.

I am grateful for Amr, in the present tense. I will not write that I "was" grateful for him because that wouldn't be the truth. I am grateful for him even now that he is not by my side. I am grateful for him because he changed me, he taught me, and he grew with me. He is still a part of my life even though we can no longer speak to or see one another. He is ever present in my heart and in my prayers.

Yes, I *am* grateful for Amr.

*****

My first meeting with Amr was completely unplanned. I traveled to Egypt with my mother for a short three-week visit in 2010 and while we were there, my uncle (who I suspect knew that I was not interested in meeting anyone) craftily brought up the topic of marriage. He told me a few things about Amr: he was twenty-three years old, a pharmacist, religious, and a long-time neighbour of my uncle. I felt that familiar wall go up inside my brain. I knew of men his age (I was nearly two years older than him) and they all seemed to be unsuitable matches for me. Although I desperately wanted to decline meeting him, I was too embarrassed to say "no" to my matchmaker uncle. To comfort myself, I thought that my meeting with Amr would become just another interesting event to add to my arsenal of bad proposal experiences.

When I entered my uncle's home to meet Amr, I was greeted by the familiar sunken couches worn down by generations of my rowdy cousins, the aroma of perpetual cooking, and the whirring of fans attempting to soften the Egyptian summer heat.

Amr hadn't arrived yet, but I saw his CV sitting on the table and I took a look at it. "What a nerd!" I humorously chuckled to myself. He had graduated with a Bachelor of Pharmacy, literally at the top of his class. I had to admit that he looked pretty good on paper. He was clearly intelligent and goal-oriented.

When he arrived, we sat nervously across from each other. I clutched my hands on my knees and felt beads of sweat forming on my forehead. My mouth felt dry and I silently hoped I wouldn't be tongue-tied. My uncle talked for a while, trying to cut the tension in the room. Amr seemed to be just as nervous as I was, fiddling with his glasses and clasping and unclasping his hands repeatedly. It made it easier for me to talk to him knowing

I wasn't the only one who felt awkward during this first meeting.

It was that day that Amr and I starting talking about everything and nothing, and I let myself notice that he had a sweet and easy smile. His eyes were searching, trying to make sense of what he was hearing and seeing. They focused under raised eyebrows when I asked puzzling questions and became pleasingly narrow when he laughed at any one of my numerous ludicrous comments. His gestures mimicked mine – a subconscious indication of interest.

When I left our first meeting that night, I was in a perplexed state. I have never believed in love at first sight; I think it's a shallow concept concocted by the entertainment industry to make love stories seem more interesting. Still, something felt different this time. Whereas I often felt relieved to be done with meeting a potential spouse, Amr's company was pleasant and I hoped that we would meet again. I was reserved in my comments and thoughts, fearing that unbridled optimism would get the better of me and I would eventually be disappointed again. I remember thinking: *This person doesn't seem like anyone I've ever met.*

And he wasn't.

In my love story I didn't love Amr at first sight. He didn't love me at first sight either. The next day, though, I received a call from my uncle telling me that Amr wanted to meet me again. When I hung up, I said to my mom, "Well of course he wants to meet me again. I'm awesome!"

She laughed and said, "Don't be so full of yourself!" I would later find out that my uncle, being the sly matchmaker that he is, called Amr and used a similar line, saying *I* wanted to meet *him* again. It's a good thing he used his mischievous tactics to get Amr and me in the same room together again. We were both too reserved to come out and say we wanted to meet each other a second time.

Amr and I met again and talked for a long time. I was traveling back to Canada the next day so it would be the last time I talked to him in person for awhile.

*****

Over the next few months, Amr and I spoke regularly online, asking each other every possible question we could think of. We were attempting to understand and appreciate each other's personalities, goals, and dreams. It didn't take us long to discover that we were two halves of one. Neither of us said it outright, but we both *knew*.

I remember my friend asking me after I had gotten engaged, "When is the exact moment you *knew* he was the one for you?"

Although our affection came on gradually, I knew the answer to that question pretty well (and the answer is quite silly). Amr had a picture of himself and his brother on Facebook that made me smile in recognition the moment I saw it. In the picture, they looked so much alike that it was as though one were a reflection of the other. They were dressed the same: smart black suits, fancy black shoes, blue dress shirts, and striped ties. They sat on their mom's couch, both making the same funny faces. When I saw that picture, I knew Amr was the one for me because I have the same "twin" picture with my sister, the two of us sitting on a bench, dressed exactly alike, our faces turned toward the camera wearing identical facial expressions.

On the surface this may seem like an odd "aha" moment to recognize that someone is meant for you, but in comparing those two pictures I instantly recognized a similar quirkiness in our personalities. How strange it was to come upon that photo one day and think: *Amr is the male version of me*. I say it's strange because I was born and raised in Canada and he was born and raised in Egypt. I would have thought there would be a significant gap in culture and understanding, but there wasn't. When someone is meant to be yours for a time, Allah (swt) causes your hearts to come together fully even if your mind initially sees barriers. What is meant to be, *is*. It's as simple as that.

My dad took into consideration his brother's (my uncle's) recommendation of Amr, but that wasn't the end of it. He conducted a thorough background check, searching high and low for people who personally knew Amr and could offer insight into his personality, values, and level of piety.

My siblings and I call my dad "the strainer" because of his uncanny skill in sifting through scores of losers to recognize men of quality for his daughters. Most men had personalities, beliefs, or traits that would never get past my dad. He would sort through them as though he had a sixth sense of who was suitable and who didn't measure up. Only a very few were considered good enough. Amr was one of them.

Once Amr and I were both comfortable enough with each other and knew that we wanted to move forward in our relationship, my father and I traveled back to Egypt together to meet Amr's family for the first time. His family was wonderful and hospitable. I still remember the elegant tray of baklava they brought when they first came to meet me and the numerous delicious and elaborate meals they painstakingly prepared whenever they hosted us. They were kind enough to overlook my nervousness and lack of both familiarity with Egyptian culture and fluency in Arabic. My dad and I were in Egypt for only six days but Amr and I met and talked often. Amr wasn't able to take that week off work so he had to work overnight shifts at the pharmacy in order to free up his days to sit and talk to me.

After much discussion between the two of us and between my father and me, plus many *istikharah* prayers, Amr and I were engaged on October 12, 2010. It was a simple meeting at Amr's parents' home without a party or celebration. My father turned to Amr's parents and asked, "Do you agree for your son to be engaged to my daughter?"

"We agree," they said.

He then turned to me and asked, "Do you agree to be engaged to Amr?"

"Yes," I nodded.

He turned to Amr.

"Do you agree to be engaged to Asmaa?"

Amr nodded solemnly. "Yes."

My father nodded. "And I agree."

That was it – simple, beautiful, *real*.

I turned to look at Amr and he was beaming. I could see he was trying to hold it in. It wasn't working, though. His smile burst from his face and he was absolutely beaming. "*Mabrook*," I said to him, grinning back. His mother caught me in a hug.

My dad and I were scheduled to leave for Canada that same night. Before we left, Amr asked me if I had brought a ring with me on this trip. He wanted to borrow it because he was going to buy me a ring before I left (he was a hopeless romantic). I let him borrow my ring so he could run off quickly to buy me one in the right size. In his words, he didn't want me to leave Egypt "empty-handed."

When we had finished packing, Amr drove us to the station in Alexandria, where we would board a bus to the Cairo airport. My dad sat in the passenger seat and I sat behind them. I looked at Amr in the rearview mirror and felt absolutely serene. There were no butterflies of nervousness or anxiety, just an inward prayer that Allah (swt) would guide us to grow into better people in one another's company.

When we arrived at the station, Amr turned to me (all while my father was still sitting next to him) and presented me with a small red velvety box.

"Asmaa, will you marry me?" he asked, grinning.

I was glad it was nighttime so he couldn't see the red flush that spread across my face. I took the box from him and opened it. It was a simple gold ring he had picked out himself. It was beautiful.

"Yes, *in sha'Allah*," I replied. I took the ring out of the box and put it on. I glanced at my father and glimpsed an embarrassed but entertained chuckle forming on his lips.

We loaded our luggage onto the bus and said our goodbyes before the bus drove off. I spent most of the time on the bus replaying every moment and conversation we had had over the past six days.

And, of course, I stared at my ring.

*****

Back in Canada, I told only a few of my close friends about the engagement. Amr and I hadn't made our news public yet. Amr absolutely loved to surprise people, so he announced our engagement on Facebook without telling his friends about me at all beforehand. We sat back and watched our profiles explode with comments from friends who were happy for us (and friends who were happy but surprised there had been no earlier hints about our engagement).

When we got engaged, Amr and I hadn't yet set the date for our *nikah*. The way our families' schedules seemed to be going at the time, we assumed the *nikah* would take place the following summer. However, neither of us wanted to have that long of an engagement because we felt it could potentially lead us to overstep Islamic boundaries. Allah (swt) made it easy for us to manage our families' schedules and we were able to get married in December, just two and a half months after we were engaged.

When my family and I traveled to Egypt in December 2010 for the *nikah*, almost all our luggage got lost. I showed up in Egypt literally with just the clothes on my back. (*Alhamdu lillah* I'd had enough sense to pack the dress I planned to wear for the *nikah* in my carry-on luggage!)

*****

December 23, 2010 was the best day of my life.

I knew getting married would be special, but I didn't like the idea of comparing it to every other day in my life as though nothing could ever match that happiness again. Until that day, I didn't understand why people said that the day you get married is the best day of your life.

The morning of December 23 was sunny, cool, and calm. I slept in, then took my time getting out of bed and eating breakfast. My then-fiancé came to pick something up from our place before the wedding and I peeked at him from the top floor of our apartment and smiled a delicious kind of secret smile. Slow conversations carried me into the afternoon, when I ironed my dress carefully, ensuring all its folds were crisp and clean.

The florist delivered my bouquet and the cake arrived as I was getting ready. I put the dress on and looked in the mirror. As I stood looking at my reflection, I felt no nerves, no doubts: just an overwhelming sense of determination. I had found *the one*. I had taken the means I had been blessed with and was marrying him. It seemed to be the most logical and easy decision I had ever made. I pinned my hijab in place.

I clanked my way to the car in my high heels, holding my dress aloft so it stayed pristine until the ceremony. We drove by the Mediterranean Sea on the way to the mosque and felt its cool winter breeze. I was chewing gum, smiling, and joking with my sisters as though I were out on a regular day, running an errand. We arrived on time and I scuttled into the mosque, making sure he didn't see me in my dress before the ceremony. I waited with my family in the women's prayer area, greeting guests and replying to the ocean of *mabrooks* being whispered into my ears.

After we finished the *'isha* prayer, I made my way up to the balcony of the mosque to have a clear view of the whole ceremony. I was the last to get up there and the women had crowded the viewing areas. With what seemed to be my sheer psychological strength, I willed them to part and soon I stood looking into the crowd of men, trying to spot the friend who was about to become my husband.

He signed and fingerprinted our marriage contract. The contract made its way upstairs so I could do the same. My writing was wobbly and lopsided but my name was clear. *I agree*, said my ink-stained thumb. I looked over the balcony railing and watched as my father sat near Amr and said the words that officially gave me away to my husband. In a moment, I was wrapped in the arms of women I knew and loved as well as women I had just met for the first time. They were ecstatic. There were many happy tears. I glanced down at the men's section and tried to scan the crowded room for Amr, but he was also lost in the arms of friends and relatives.

I felt the same as I had before I was married: happy, calm, sure of myself. It seemed like nothing had changed.

My husband escaped the grips of his enthusiastic friends and made his way up to the women's section to exchange rings with me. His face was bright and filled with an innocent bewilderment as he took my hand and kissed my forehead (to the soundtrack of giggling women). My cheeks were flushed but it all seemed like the most natural sequence of events – as if I had somehow known beforehand that it was going to happen this way.

Chocolates and drinks were passed around. I didn't get a chance to taste them. My husband saved a chocolate for me to eat later but my brother got to it first. And that was okay.

We linked arms and made our way out of the mosque to be greeted by a crowd of happy faces, confetti, and hand-held fireworks. My husband's friends ambushed him, hoisted him up, and threw him up into the air a few times. I looked on in amusement and kept stealing glances at this man who was now my closest partner in life. I smiled because I absolutely knew he was the right ally to make. After snapping some photos, Amr took me by the hand and led me from the festivities to his friend's car to drive us away.

Between the smiles and careful, treasured first words, I quietly said, *"Alhamdu lillah."* I knew that I would never again be surprised by anything beautiful that Allah allowed me to have in my life. He was the only One capable of bringing two people from different parts of the globe together – people who didn't know about each other just a year before, people who weren't even interested in love anymore, people who had surrendered themselves to the harshness of disappointment.

But Allah is *al-Fattah*, the Opener of doors, opportunities, and chances to regain piety, forgiveness, and love. Nothing more remains for me except to thank Him every day for making what seemed to be so hard at first so easy and wonderful, full of immense beauty and contentment.

Now I understand why people say getting married is the best day of your life. It's true.

Alhamdu lillah.

Losing Amr

Marrying and living with Amr was like finally seeing the sun rise over the landscape of my heart after a long, dark, cold night. Losing him was not peaceful like the setting sun, though. It was terrifying and painful. It was as though that radiant sun were being destroyed, piece-by-piece, in front of my eyes.

We had a happy life together and a nine-month-old daughter when Amr was taken. Our time together was so short, as though it were just a passing dream.

After we married I moved to Egypt, where we lived for a little over a year. It was in that year that I first garnered the courage to venture out alone into Egypt's haphazard chaos. I learned how to take creaky microbuses on my own and to maneuver so I would not sit next to strange men on my travels. It was in that year that I first learned how to cook. I messed up quite a bit when Amr was my unfortunate taste-test subject, but he never once complained. It was in that year that I learned the positive and negative idiosyncrasies of Egyptian culture.

It was also in that year that I witnessed firsthand Amr's remarkable character. He prayed every prayer in the mosque. He fasted every Monday and Thursday as well as the three middle days of each lunar calendar month. He was incredibly kind and generous. He insisted that everything that was *his* was now *mine*, too.

Prior to moving to Egypt, I had applied to sponsor Amr to come to Canada as a permanent resident. When we finally got the news that he had been approved, we were excited to start a new chapter in our lives together. Amr had shown me all the places he loved in Egypt; now it was my turn to show him all the places I loved when I was growing up in Toronto.

Moving to a new country was hard for Amr. He spoke English fluently but Canadian culture was so different from what he was accustomed to. Still, he got up every morning and did whatever was in his power to provide for his family and open up new opportunities for us.

By the time we arrived in Canada, I was already four months pregnant. Amr was working part time and applying for Master's degree programs at different universities. Much of his time was devoted to fleshing out his different study and work options and doing some research work with a professor at a nearby university.

A few months later we had our baby. She was born on November 10, 2012 in the same Toronto hospital where I had been born twenty-six years earlier. After nine months of the two of us thinking our baby was a boy, she was born and the doctor plainly pronounced, "It's a girl." They handed her to me. After all the hours of labour there she was: a six-pound, five-ounce piece of perfection. We called her Ruqaya.

We dove headfirst into the exhaustion and sleepless nights of parenting. For the next few months, Ruqaya's feedings, diaper changes, teething, and doctor's visits were all that occupied me.

*****

Amr and I decided to travel to Egypt in June 2013 so his parents could meet their granddaughter for the first time.

We booked our flights and were preoccupied with packing and arranging everything for our trip.

The summer of 2013 was a tumultuous time to be in Egypt, to say the least. When we traveled to Egypt in early June, we were completely unaware of how serious and dangerous the situation on the ground would become.

Large protests were taking place against the Muslim Brotherhood-led government. On July 3, 2013, a few weeks after we arrived in the country, we witnessed the removal of the first democratically-elected president, Mohamed Morsi, in a coup d'état led by the Egyptian military. The president and his aides were arrested and soon counter-protests calling for Morsi's reinstatement started cropping up, leading to mass encampments and sit-ins by his supporters. What emerged in the days and weeks that followed was a wave of rampant injustices committed by the military, leading up to what is described by Human Rights Watch as "one of the world's largest killings of demonstrators in a single day in recent history" at Rabaa Square in Cairo on August 14, 2013. In the two months that followed the coup, over 1,150 innocent men, women, and children were killed in cold blood, the majority of them in Rabaa Square.[1]

Needless to say, throughout the weeks following the coup, our worries increased. We had planned to fly back to Toronto on August 19, but Allah (swt) had planned something else for our small family.

On August 16, 2013, two days after the Rabaa Massacre in Cairo, Amr was at a large protest in Alexandria. He clearly understood the injustice of the military coup and its serious ramifications. He was devastated at the murder of hundreds of protesters just two days prior and had joined this local protest to stand up for the rights of his brothers and sisters who had been killed indiscriminately.

Amr never shied away from speaking the truth. August 16 was no different. That afternoon, I called Amr to make sure he was okay and to ask when he would be home. He quelled my fears, told me he was on his way home, and assured me that everything was fine. He said there had been thousands of people at the protest: men, women, and children. I asked him to pick up diapers for Ruqaya on his way home. He laughed and said, "Okay."

I told him I loved him.

That was our last conversation.

About twenty minutes later, I received a call from Amr's number. When I answered, an unfamiliar voice was on the other end. I handed the phone to my mother-in-law because I didn't understand what the man on the phone was saying. He told her that Amr had been martyred and that passersby at the protest had carried his body to a nearby mosque. He said someone from Amr's family should come take possession of his body.

Our initial reaction was one of shock. We didn't know whether to believe the news or not. I felt a heavy knot tying itself in my stomach. Before any tears came, I eyed the washroom sink, thinking that I would throw up at any moment. Amr's parents were in hysterics. His father quickly ran out of the apartment to make his way to the mosque where Amr's body was supposed to be. We didn't tell anyone for an hour or so; we had to verify the news of

Amr's murder before I could even call my parents. It was a long, difficult hour. Soon we received a call from Amr's father: it really was Amr's body in the mosque's makeshift morgue. His soul was gone.

Around forty-five others were killed in the same place on that same day.

The minutes, days, and weeks that followed were the most difficult, darkest moments of my life. I was caught between the immense pain of losing my partner and the urgency of trying to figure out how to safely leave the country with Ruqaya.

In the days after Amr's martyrdom, I kept looking at my beautiful, unaffected daughter and thinking: *You are an orphan now.* I kept looking at myself in the mirror and thinking: *You are a widow now.* When I tried to look into my future, I couldn't see a single thing. Everything I had planned for my life, I had planned with Amr. Suddenly, none of those plans were relevant anymore.

One of the most frightening experiences is to look forward into your life and see nothing: no happiness, no hope, no potential. In that blindness, the only thing I could hear was my own heart, rattling towards what seemed like a future of hollow nothingness. I couldn't imagine ever recovering from that pain.

I *had* to recover, though. I had to be happy again for my daughter's sake. I had to learn how to live in the presence of death without being paralyzed by it.

And, by the permission of Allah, I did learn to get up and walk forward again.

This is my journey: a journey that has been filled with a kind of pain I never knew existed, but also a depth of serenity and gratitude that was new, deep, and beautiful.

The journal entries on the following pages are short records I kept of the highs and lows I endured in the two years following Amr's departure from this world. Writing was a way for me to process my pain and attempt to emerge from it with a greater understanding of my faith and of myself. Some of these entries are reflections I shared on social media platforms because I felt the pressing need to tell my story to everyone who would listen. I needed the world to know about Amr.

In this book are words that have given me comfort and have reminded me that beyond the pain and darkness of loss there is still the potential of light in patience and constancy.

{O mankind, there has to come to you instruction from your Lord and healing for what is in the breasts and guidance and mercy for the believers.}   *(Yoonus 10:57)*

ʻIddah

Four months and ten days

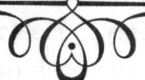

August 18, 2013

{Think not of those who are killed in the way of Allah as dead. Nay, they are alive, with their Lord, and they have provision.

They rejoice in what Allah has bestowed upon them of His bounty, rejoicing for the sake of those who have not yet joined them, but are left behind (not yet martyred) that on them no fear shall come, nor shall they grieve.

They rejoice in a grace and a bounty from Allah, and that Allah will not waste the reward of the believers.}

(Âl-'Imrân 3:169-171)

My husband, Amr Mohamed Kassem, was twenty-six years old when he returned to his Lord on Friday, August 16, 2013 after the *'asr* prayer. He was shot through his chin and the bullet exited at the back of his neck. He was at a protest in Alexandria, calling for justice for all those who had been killed mercilessly all over Egypt by the army in the previous days and weeks.

Yesterday morning I went to the morgue at a nearby hospital in Alexandria to see Amr before he would be washed and buried a few hours later. When I arrived, there were many people waiting outside the doors to see their own family members as numerous people were killed the same day as Amr. Some of Amr's friends and relatives were there, too. After waiting awhile, I entered the room where his body was lying on a table, covered by a long blanket.

I stood beside him and uncovered his face. There he was – my love – lying cold even though I had seen him strong, happy, and smiling just twenty-four hours earlier. I stroked his beard. Part of it was still soft, but part was hardened with dried blood. His nose was bloodied and he had a cut beside his eye but he was beautiful, even in death: silent as though sleeping. I touched his lips and his cheeks. They were cold.

I stood for some time looking at his face, feeling as though my heart were being repeatedly run over by a truck. I refused to cry loudly but tears were streaming down my cheeks. I whispered to him, "I love you, Amr. I know that you always wanted to die for the sake of Allah and you got what you always hoped for, *in sha'Allah*. I'm so proud of you."

Then I made the most difficult *du'a* I have ever made: "*Ya Allah!* Forgive his sins and accept him as a martyr. Reunite me with him in the hereafter. *Ya Allah!* Make me patient in knowing that it was his appointed time and that, by Your will and grace, he is alive with You as a martyr."

I didn't leave him until I was ready. I'm not sure how long I was standing there. At the end, I kissed his cheek and told him that I would see him later. I covered his face and left the room.

The funeral was after the *'asr* prayer on Saturday. Hundreds of people were there: his friends, his colleagues from school and work, and both of our extended families. He was a beloved person to many. There was not a dry eye in the crowd but everyone was speaking only good words and saying *alhamdu lillah* that Allah took him in one of the best ways anyone can die. We performed the funeral prayer, then I went outside to see a crowd of hundreds of men carrying Amr's shrouded body quickly towards the cemetery. The women didn't follow right away. We were waiting until he was buried before we went to his grave.

After some time, his mother and I walked into the cemetery with some female relatives, making our way to where he was buried. Suddenly, I noticed all the men around me yelling for us to find a side gate to escape the cemetery. I heard loud shouting and bangs behind me from rocks being thrown at us. The men who were a part of Amr's funeral were yelling at the women to run.

As I ran without looking back, I was struck on my cheek with a large rock. Some of Amr's friends saw me and told me to run ahead of them so they could make sure nothing happened to me. The people who attacked us were almost certainly state-sponsored thugs who showed up to cause trouble upon hearing there was a "Muslim Brotherhood" funeral taking place.[2] Many people were injured, some with stab wounds, but there were no casualties, *alhamdu lillah*.

Even in death, Amr's enemies hated him and all those around him! Their hate means nothing to me, though. After all, if an enemy of Allah hates you then that is a sign that you are, *in sha'Allah*, on the right path.

Dear friends, my heart aches in a way I never knew a heart could ache. I miss him whenever I'm awake and dream about him when I'm asleep. He was the best husband a woman could ever hope for: kind, generous, soft, and loving but also strong and brave. His clothes are still hung up in our room as though he's going to walk through the door and change into his pajamas before he sleeps.

Through all this, I can't say anything except *inna lillahi wa inna ilayhi raji'oon* – to Allah we belong and to

Him we will return – and continue to make *du'a* for him. I refuse to dishonour him or myself by asking Allah why he took Amr or thinking: *If only he hadn't gone to the protest on Friday, he would be alive.*

It was Amr's time to return to Allah; I know that beyond a shadow of a doubt. Although I wish I'd had more time with him in this world, I sincerely look forward to reuniting with him and being his wife, if Allah allows me, in paradise. In the hereafter time does not end and there is no fear of being separated from your loved ones. I believe with every inch of my being that our love was truly a love that can last from this world to the next.

Last night after we came home, we received a call from a friend of a relative who had witnessed firsthand what had happened to Amr after he was shot. She told us that he didn't die right away; he was alive for a few moments. His left hand held his chin where the bullet had entered and his right index finger rose up as he said clearly, *"Ash-hadu an la illaha ill-Allah, wa ash-hadu anna Muhammadun rasool-ullah."*[3] He had a huge smile on his face, as though it were his wedding day. When I heard this, I couldn't help but cry tears of joy. Allah had honoured me by allowing me to be this man's wife and the mother of his child.

I ask Allah to let me never stray from His path, for my own sake and my daughter's, but also for Amr's sake: to honour him in the way Allah chose for him to leave this world.

Amr, my love: I hope that right now your soul is in a green bird and you are flying through paradise, eating and drinking from its provisions and are close to the throne of

Allah, where you will never shed another tear or ever feel any sense of loss or suffering.[4] You are my love in this world and the next, *in sha'Allah*. You are in my heart always. You are in my prayers always.

Ya Allah! You reunited Moosa's mother with him after she put him in the river.

Ya Allah! You reunited Ya'qoob with his beloved son, Yoosuf, after many years of painful separation.

Ya Allah! You are the only One Who can reunite me with my beloved in the hereafter, so I ask You to grant us an eternal life together in paradise.

August 20, 2013

"A man asked the Messenger of Allah (saws): What is the most virtuous struggle (jihad)?

The Prophet (saws) said: A word of truth in front of a tyrannical ruler."[5]

Amr's great struggle was speaking the truth in front of those who were oppressing the people. May Allah accept his struggle and grant him forgiveness and limitless mercy.

Some people have asked me why Amr's burial was delayed for an entire day. He was killed right after *'asr* prayer on Friday and buried after *'asr* prayer the next day. Twenty-four hours doesn't seem long, but usually a Muslim's funeral takes place quickly, sometimes just hours after he or she passes away (especially in a Muslim-majority country where suitable burial services are easy to access).

I wish there were a short and simple answer, but there isn't one.

After Amr was killed, other protesters quickly carried his body and took cover in a mosque nearby called Masjid 'Ali ibn Abi Talib. The people who carried his body didn't know Amr, but they refused to leave his body abandoned in the street.

After we got the call that Amr had been killed, his father, his uncle, and his brother all rushed to that mosque to see if they could help him or at least identify him. Amr's soul was already gone when they arrived. I stayed back with Amr's mom and Ruqaya. The situation was too dangerous for us to go ourselves.

Since Amr's brother works at a hospital, they thought it would be the safest place to take him until they could figure out what to do next. Amr was carried to the car. His body was lying across the laps of his uncle and his father. His blood stained the car's upholstery and all their clothes. While they were driving, armed men loyal to the state were looking into all the passing cars; when they saw that Amr was bearded, they began to attack the car. His soul was already gone, but they couldn't even let his body go in peace! They banged on the car with pipes and weapons and even shot a bullet at the car.

Amr's uncle covered Amr's beard so that the thugs they were passing in the street wouldn't see what he looked like. Amr's brother finally sped away. No one else was hurt, *alhamdu lillah*.

By the time they arrived at the hospital morgue, it was close to the time for the *'isha* prayer. After doing some paperwork for Amr's death certificate, the men returned home and left Amr there overnight.

None of us slept that night.

The next morning, Amr's mom and I went to see his body and say goodbye. The coroner was the next person in. It was only after his examination that we learned Amr had been shot through the chin (we previously thought he had been shot through the back of his neck but that was actually where the bullet had exited his body). We initially couldn't see the entry wound on his chin because his thick beard was covering it.

We set the time of the funeral for after *'asr* prayer to allow for the coroner's visit as well as the washing of Amr's body.

I was preoccupied with the fact that I wasn't with Amr in his final moments. I kept wondering: *What pains did he feel? What thoughts ran through his mind in those few seconds after he was shot? Did he suffer much?*

I was reminded today, though, of this hadith of the Prophet (saws):

"A martyr only feels from the effect of being killed that which one would feel when being stung by a mosquito."[6]

I pray that Amr is counted among the martyrs. I pray that he didn't suffer or feel any pain. I pray that Allah (swt) blesses him with complete joy and serenity that instantly makes up for every tear and ounce of pain he ever felt in this world.

August 23, 2013

My soul, you would never mourn a bird that was released from its cage and now roams freely in the heavens. So, too, should you contain your mourning for your beloved one now that he is free.

August 24, 2013

It has been one week since Amr was buried and today I was able to visit his grave for the first time. I went with his parents, his brother, and Ruqaya. The graveyard was strangely silent compared to all the noise and commotion of the surrounding city.

A man led us to where Amr was buried. As we followed him, I quietly recited the *du'a* of visiting the graves:

"Peace be upon you all, O inhabitants of the graves, amongst the believers and the Muslims. Indeed we are, Allah willing, soon to follow. We ask Allah for well-being for us and for you."[7]

In that moment I was aware that soon – very soon – I would be the one buried in a graveyard somewhere, being visited by my loved ones.

We arrived at Amr's grave. There was no tombstone with his name, no special markings yet, nothing to indicate that the person beneath the ground here was Amr. We stood silently, each caught up in our own thoughts, each making our own *du'as*. I asked Allah (swt) to envelop Amr in His forgiveness and mercy.

We didn't stay long.

As we rode in a taxi back to my in-laws' home, I felt a sense of relief overcome me. Everything was final. Everything was settled. I had to see Amr's grave before leaving Egypt, as though I needed to make sure he was really gone.

He was really gone and it was time to go home.

August 26, 2013

Ruqaya and I are back in Canada. For the entire week after Amr was killed, my family in Toronto had been trying to arrange an appropriate flight for us to return home, to restore some semblance of safety in our lives.

Yesterday morning on the way to the airport we drove through Alexandria. I stared out the car window, watching people hurrying from one errand to the next in the heat of the Egyptian sun. I didn't understand how they were all just going about their business as though nothing had changed, as though it were any normal day. It wasn't a normal day for me.

Soon I was standing at the airport with Amr's parents. They walked us to the sliding doors but were not allowed to continue past that point. I cannot explain in words what grief I witnessed on their faces as we said our goodbyes. Amr's father had told me just the day before, "When you and Ruqaya are here with us, I feel as though Amr is going to walk through the front door at any moment."

They hugged Ruqaya and me. I left them standing there, watching us leave: watching all they had left of their son walk off into the distance.

*****

Traveling with a nine-month-old isn't easy, but I was barely focused on that. I spent my three flights replaying everything that had happened in the last ten days and simultaneously trying to numb my emotions so I could take care of Ruqaya. After two stopovers we finally landed in

Toronto. It was strange to see the airport again. It was the airport that Amr and I had traveled from just two months earlier. We left as three but we came back as two.

I went through customs, collected my luggage, and headed to the arrival gate. It was past midnight at this point. My parents and siblings were waiting for me. I was glad to see faces that belonged to people I knew were on my side, no matter what. I hugged each of them. I didn't cry, not because I didn't want to but because I didn't have it in me. I was exhausted.

We piled into the car and drove home.

August 27, 2013

Let the dust settle at your feet. Don't remove the grains of sand from your shoes because that's the sand from the graveyard. It lines the insides of your soles. Let the sadness settle in, let it find the parts of your heart it hasn't yet touched simply because *there was no time*. Let it invade. Let it be as though you have never felt happiness before. Then let it go.

Let your husband's perfume sit on the shelf in your closet so your daughter can know how he smelled. Let his slippers lie in front of the bathroom so you can make *wudoo* in them. Read from his pocket-sized Qur'an. Look through his wallet and remember the times he got his driver's license and library card. Wear his wedding band and smile at the thought of the two of you picking it out together.

See the gold-coloured half-moon in the sky and believe the other half will return to complete it soon.

August 30, 2013

During our time in Canada, Amr struggled to find full-time, reliable employment. He had such high aspirations and was motivated to build his experience and education. Unfortunately, he was often disappointed by all the unnecessary hurdles he had to jump over to provide for his family.

He never knew, but I always used to make a special *du'a* for him.

I used to ask *al-Fattah*, the Opener, to open the doors of success for him. He opened for Amr the greatest door, leading to the greatest success in the hereafter (by His permission).

I used to ask Allah to help Amr not only achieve but also exceed his goals and leave a lasting legacy for the Muslim community. Truly, He allowed Amr to surpass his aspirations and leave a legacy for his daughter and, I hope, others as well.

I used to ask *al-Hafidh*, the Protector, to protect Amr. He protected Amr's soul from the great trials and difficulties we are currently living in.

Allah is *al-Mujeeb*, the One Who responds:

{And your Lord says: Call upon Me; I will respond to you...} *(Ghâfir 40:60)*

September 7, 2013

I have good days and bad days. My mind comprehends that Allah (swt) has a better plan for me than I could possibly have for myself. It's my heart, though, that is having a hard time understanding how to hold and process all of this pain without bursting.

I recently came upon this quote by Ibn Al-Qayyim.[8] It's a note to myself for when I don't understand Allah's plan for me:

> Had Allah lifted the veil for his slave and shown him how He handles his affairs for him, and how Allah is keener for the benefit of the slave than his own self, his heart would have melted out of the love for Allah and would have been torn to pieces out of thankfulness to Allah. Therefore if the pains of this world tire you, do not grieve. For it may be that Allah wishes to hear your voice by way of *du'a*. So pour out your desires in prostration and forget about it and know that verily Allah does not forget.

I immediately feel lighter when I raise my hands to Allah (swt) and admit my pain and need to Him. It's as though I am depositing all my sadness and fears into His care, knowing that He will soon relieve my sorrows, knowing that He will never forget me. How merciful and loving He is to His slaves!

September 11, 2013

Our story has reached many parts of the world. People from every continent have read about me and Amr. Now I find myself sifting through hundreds of private messages and comments on social media where people praise me in ways that are not reflective of reality. I wish people would stop telling me that I'm strong, patient, and inspirational.

If they could reach into the depth of my pain, they wouldn't say I was strong. If they could see just the edges of my sadness, they wouldn't say I was patient. If they could touch the ache in my heart, they wouldn't say I was inspirational.

Every day I have to remind myself that Allah (swt) created me as a human. I'm not an angel made from light. I'm just a human, made from the clay of the earth.

The earth quakes, as does my heart. The earth changes and is flooded and is cracked open. It is snowed and rained upon. It dies and is brought back to life. It can be beautiful and it can be frightening.

Above all, the earth is never just one thing. I am also never just one thing.

I write and share because that is how I survive. To write is to purge myself of this strange darkness within me, examine its shape and colour and taste so that I can attempt to transform it into hope.

And now, more than ever, I need to hope.

September 14, 2013

I am coming home,
with black and red seeping through my skin,
with clouded senses and a vague numbness.

I am coming home,
your wedding band and daughter in hand.

Nights have passed, and mornings have passed.
There has been rain and sun and wind
and my heart was made public with grief for the
    loss of your smell
and your hands and your laugh.

But I am coming home
to where blood is not spilled, children not orphaned,
    hearts not trampled.

Wait for me by the edge, perhaps we can talk into eternity.

September 15, 2013

Life has its distractions, but the moment always comes when I find myself alone with my thoughts and memories and it feels as though there's nothing to keep me from drowning in sadness over what I've lost. At that point the only thing that keeps my head above water is the remembrance of Allah.

Don't ever underestimate Allah's words:

{...Verily in the remembrance of Allah do hearts find rest.}   *(ar-Ra'd 13:28)*

Turning to Him through prayer, *du'a*, or reading His words is the only true solace I've found for my grieving heart.

The person I loved most is gone, but the Lord who listens best is still here.

September 18, 2013

My Lord! Your slave, Amr, brought joy and light into the hearts of so many people around him, so bring joy and light into his grave.

My Lord! Your slave was restless on this earth, always trying to find ways to please You and take care of his family, so give him a beautiful and peaceful rest.

My Lord! Your slave took care of the ties of kinship, so take care of him and grant him Your forgiveness.

My Lord! Your slave looked upon his wife and daughter with love and mercy, so love him and look upon him with Your mercy.

My Lord! Open the doors of paradise to him and fill his grave with cool breeze, brightness, and perfumes.

My Lord! You are the Patient, so grant us the patience to accept the departure of our beloved.

Ameen.

September 30, 2013

When I am about to lose myself in grief, I remember the verse:

{On no soul does Allah place a burden greater than it can bear...} *(al-Baqarah 2:286)*

I know that my Lord is the Most Merciful and He has already given me the strength, the bravery, and the patience to overcome. Now it's up to me to discover, understand, and employ that strength.

October 2, 2013

Sadness doesn't have to be a big, gaping hole. It can be a trip to buy just one coffee, laundry for two instead of three, and silence instead of conversation.

The quiet ways of loneliness are the hardest. May Allah (swt) relieve our loneliness by granting us eternal companionship with those we love in paradise.

Our eyes shed tears and our hearts are filled with grief, but we do not say anything except that by which Allah is pleased.[9]

October 5, 2013

In the days and weeks that followed Amr's departure from this world, I reached deep within myself and extracted a kind of *du'a* that I had never made before: a *du'a* of complete need, a *du'a* of complete surrender, a *du'a* of someone who was oppressed.

The *du'a* of desperation is not like any other. Nothing can decrease my pain except the tears that stream down my cheeks as I ask Allah (swt) to grant me justice against Amr's killers and to grant me patience and strength to be the woman and mother that I need to be.

My Lord, I leave the oppressors to You. Deal with them in a manner befitting Your justice. Leave none of them on this earth except that he or she is plagued with misery and disease until the day they meet You and wish they were made into dust.

People often tell me that to forgive someone who has wronged me is better, that it is truly the higher manifestation of faith. But today I am human. Today I am oppressed. Today I need, more than anything in the world, to make the *du'a* that I am entitled to make.

Anas ibn Malik (ra) reported that the Messenger of Allah (saws) said:

"Beware of the supplication of the oppressed, for there is no screen between it and Allah."[10]

October 6, 2013

A few weeks ago we were being chased by armed thugs after Amr was buried. I couldn't believe that I was running for my life in a graveyard.

Upon reflection, Allah (swt) showed me a frightening reality that day: we are all walking or running through graveyards, towards the spots we will be buried in. We just don't know it yet.

October 9, 2013

Amr loved nature. It was one of his favourite things about Canada. The overpopulated concrete cities of Egypt that he was accustomed to were no comparison to the open spaces and lush gardens of Toronto's parks.

When I miss him I say, *"Subhan Allahul-'Adheem wa bihamdihi* (glory and praise be to Allah, the Almighty)." Each time a believer says this phrase, a palm tree is planted for him or her in paradise.[11]

If Allah grants me the opportunity to meet Amr again in paradise and our home is surrounded by vast palm tree groves, he'll know I planted those for him, *in sha'Allah.*

October 16, 2013

I have come to realize in the last two months that *husn adh-dhann billah* (having a good opinion of Allah) is one of the most important things to live by, both in times of hardship and in times of ease.

When Allah tested our family with the loss of our most loved friend, brother, son, and husband – our Amr – we believed that Allah took him out of His mercy to shield him from the hurt of further trials.

We believe that Allah has forgiven him and honoured him.

We believe that He wants us to turn to Him in repentance and *du'a* so that He can forgive and honour us, too.

We believe that perhaps Allah loves us and this is a means for Him to count us among those who are patient.

We believe that his parents will have the House of Praise in paradise for their pain and patience.[12]

We believe that much good will come to the world from his life and death.

We believe that He will reunite us with Amr in the hereafter.

This is *al-Jabbar*, the Compeller, mending us and carrying our hearts forward.

{And (remember) Ayyoob, when he cried to his Lord: Verily, distress has seized me, and You are the Most Merciful of all those who show mercy.

So We answered his call, and We removed the distress that was on him, and We restored his family to him (that he had lost), and the like thereof along with them, as a mercy from Ourselves and a reminder for all who worship Us.}

(al-Anbiyâ' 21:83-84)

October 20, 2013

When Amr passed into the next world, he left behind every material possession that normally he never would have been without: his wallet, his ID, his money, his clothes, his wedding band. He went into the grave with no weapon or armour except his good deeds.

Prophet Muhammad (saws) said:

"When carried to his grave, a dead person is followed by three, two of which return (after his burial) and one of which remains with him: his relatives, his property, and his deeds follow him; his relatives and his property go back while his deeds remain with him."[13]

Perhaps this is not a new observation, but when I think deeply about this I am shaken; we are left mourning over him and all we have left are his *things*. I swear by Allah, I would give every single dollar I own and every material thing I have if it meant I could see his smile just one more time.

It has taken me the greatest loss to truly understand that whether you are alive or dead, material possessions are absolutely worthless. They don't give you what your heart really needs in this world, nor do they come to your aid once you have died.

Remove the love of material possessions from your heart and give away everything you can afford. Save yourself from hell even if it is by giving just half a date in charity.[14]

October 24, 2013

When I look into my mother's eyes, I see the sorrow that she hides and the desire to do anything to take the pain from my heart. When I look into my daughter's eyes, I wish that I, too, could take any pain away from her, even before it happens.

A mother's love is unlike any other. It's uncomplicated, pure, unselfish, unconditional. When my daughter cries, I go to her. When she gives me a hard time, I forgive her and love her anyway. When she smiles, my whole world in that moment is bright and beautiful.

Allah is more merciful to His believing slaves than any mother is to her child.[15] If we come back to Him after we fall, He will embrace us. If we cry in pain to Him, He will soothe us. If we ask to be guided, He will guide us.

He always gives us exactly what we need, even if we don't understand it.

October 26, 2013

What disturbs me most about indiscriminate killing, whether it's in Egypt or elsewhere, is that the person doing the killing must have a mother, a father, a child, or a spouse he loves dearly.

Doesn't he rely on someone every day? Doesn't he look forward to meeting him or her? Doesn't he revel in the beauty and serenity of being held by someone he loves?

Of course he does.

So how could he take away someone's life so easily when that person is a mother, a father, a child, and someone's love? How could he pull a trigger and end the joy of so many people at once and not imagine how he would feel if someone did the same to him?

How dark must one's heart be to cause all this damage?

If we become complacent viewers of this evil, our humanity suffers and *our* hearts become dark, too.

October 27, 2013

Allah (swt) is merciful. Even in my difficulty, He often grants me moments of absolute contentment and serenity. It is during these moments that I become aware of Allah's power in that I understand there is no enemy too strong for Him to conquer, no sadness too deep for Him to alleviate, no burden too heavy for Him to lift. How free from imperfection He is!

October 28, 2013

Earlier this year Amr was working at a pharmacy here in Toronto. Yesterday, my dad went into the pharmacy to buy something and was approached by one of Amr's former co-workers, an older Somali woman. She wanted to offer her condolences.

This woman stood weeping in front of my father out of sadness for having lost the kind co-worker she once knew. Even though it has been two and a half months since Amr departed, his character is still surprising me every day. It seems there is no person he met whose heart he didn't touch in some way or another.

I didn't realize that Amr was not only my husband, but also my teacher.

We impact every person we meet in either a positive or negative way, even if at first we don't realize it. We sometimes forget that part of the beauty of Islam lies in the beauty of character. Our Prophet (saws) was a man of unsurpassed character. He spread mercy, peace, and truth everywhere he went and everywhere he was known.

Good character will cause those around you to love you, to want to always be near you, to want to be better people, and to remember you in their supplications.

May Allah (swt) forgive Amr, love him, and enter him into the highest levels of paradise. May Allah (swt) bless us with a beautiful legacy after we pass away and make our lives a means of spreading only good in the world.

October 30, 2013

When Ruqaya sees a picture of her dad she smiles and reaches out towards him, opening and closing her hand. She wants him to come. Right then, when my heart is about to burst for my cherub, I remember that Allah (swt) tells us:

{...But perhaps you hate a thing and it is good for you; and perhaps you love a thing and it is bad for you. And Allah knows, while you know not.}　　　　*(al-Baqarah 2:216)*

Perhaps Allah wishes good for our small family. Perhaps He is purifying us and calling us to Him through this pain. Perhaps when Ruqaya is all grown up, I will tell her that this difficulty caused my heart to become disconnected from this world and it should only make us work harder and longer to reach our home near Him.

November 1, 2013

Amr rarely went anywhere without his pocket-sized Qur'an. Ruqaya, who has been fascinated with books since she was born, would inevitably end up in his lap trying her best to grab it and "read" with him.

On a few occasions in Egypt he would accidentally leave these small copies of the Qur'an behind in the different places he went. He always bought another one right away so he wouldn't be without it.

Perhaps those copies that he left behind have found their way into the hands and hearts of others who love the Qur'an as much as he did.

I now hold his last pocket-sized Qur'an in my hands and in my heart. It only cost him a few Egyptian pounds to purchase, but it has become my most prized possession.

May Allah (swt) allow the Qur'an to intercede for him and for us on the Final Day.

November 3, 2013

Sometimes the sadness seems like it will take over. It feels as though no matter what good and beautiful things happen in my life, they can't possibly replace what I've lost. Then I read this and I know that the only sadness that is forever is the sadness that comes from not knowing Allah:

Truly in the heart there is a sadness that cannot be removed except with the happiness of knowing Allah and being true to Him. And in it there is an emptiness that cannot be filled except with love for Him and by turning to Him and always remembering Him. And if a person were given all of the world and what is in it, it would not fill this emptiness.

And verily for everything that a slave loses there is a substitute, but the one who loses Allah will never find anything to replace Him.   *(Ibn al-Qayyim)*

November 4, 2013

My grandfather passed away suddenly a few months ago in late May. I remember visiting Egypt in my childhood with my parents and five siblings and staying with him and my grandmother for a few weeks at a time. We would open his fridge and turn our noses up at the smelly cheeses he liked. We would run back and forth in his apartment with our cousins, barely understanding what they were saying to us in Arabic. We once hid his cigarettes because we didn't want him to smoke anymore (he did eventually stop smoking and I like to think it had something to do with our childhood insistence).

I recall his hoarse laughter and roughly-shaved face that would scrape against my skin as I kissed him on the cheek once, twice, three times. He was the centre of our family, holding onto my mother's memories and ours: the ones we didn't even know we had.

I had lost three of my grandparents before him and losing him felt like I lost a part of my history. The first thing I did when I found out was go to Amr and throw myself into his chest. I made his shirt wet with my tears.

When Amr passed away just a few months later, I found that I couldn't throw myself into anyone's chest. No one's shirt was wet with my tears except my own. I was held by many people; some I knew and some I didn't. Their arms weren't home to the warmth and love my heart craved, though. I was without an anchor in dark, stormy seas. I was alone. Losing Amr meant that I lost a part of myself. The old version of me went into the ground with him.

No matter how much I tried to explain this to people, no one knew the contents of my heart. No one understood the emptiness I saw before me when I tried to look into my future. That loneliness is not something words can describe.

I know now that Allah was teaching me in those moments that it wasn't human beings that I needed. Not a single soul knows what I know or feels exactly as I feel. He is the All-Knowing, so He knows better than anyone what my heart struggles with each day. He is the All-Seeing, so He sees what I hide away from the world. He is the All-Hearing, so He hears all my desperate pleas in the darkness of night.

From the little I know about Allah, I am satisfied. His promises are the absolute truth. If I do not leave Him, He is the only One Who will never leave me.

What better friend or companion could I possibly have?

November 6, 2013

About a week before Amr passed away, we went shopping and he bought a dark grey shirt. At the time, neither of us knew that he would be wearing that shirt when he was killed.

We may already own the clothes we are going to die in.

I know that everything comes at its time and perhaps it may take someone years to have the courage or stamina to practice Islam as he or she should. While I respect each person's journey, I now feel the urgency in not waiting. I can't wait on mending ties of kinship until it's more "convenient." I can't wait on praying properly or dressing more modestly or going for hajj until after I retire. I can't wait on giving charity until I have more to give.

I fear the moment I will be alone in my grave with nothing to shield me from my fate but my deeds. I fear that in that darkness, in my ultimate hour of need, I'll say to myself: *If only I had done more good and less evil...*

I beg of you, my soul: please don't wait. Your chance may never come.

November 10, 2013

Amr and I were having a boy – at least that's what my early ultrasound *sort of* indicated. We tried to get a clearer picture of the baby's gender later on in my pregnancy, but the baby's legs were always crossed. That's why we just thought *she* was a *he*.

Amr and I discussed baby names for months. I had my favourite names and he had his. In the end, we decided on two names: Bilal and Ruqaya. They were the only two names we could both agree on. In any case, we only picked Ruqaya as a backup name because we still thought we were having a boy.

November 10, 2012 – one year ago today – our lives changed forever. After months of thinking our baby was a boy, we were floored when the doctor casually announced, "It's a girl." Strangely, the first thing I thought was: *But all her clothes are blue!*

The day Ruqaya made her grand entrance into the world, we went from a family of two to a family of three. Amr's eyes were glowing with pride and love for this new little human who had entered our lives.

We are now back to a family of two, but we still praise Allah for His blessings on us. *Alhamdu lillah* for what we know that He has given us and *alhamdu lillah* for all He has given to us that we don't know yet or are unable to perceive due to our limited knowledge.

May your face glow, my Amr, with pride and love and gratefulness to Your Lord on the Day of Resurrection.

May the three of us be reunited under His shade.

November 11, 2013

When I first picked up the Qur'an after Amr was killed, I realized that for all the years before, I had taken the Qur'an for granted. I believed in it, I wished to memorize from it, understand it, and follow it. However, I hadn't understood how much I needed it to actually *live*. I hadn't understood that it was more important for me to know Allah through the Qur'an than it was to breathe or have a pulse.

There are days when I don't want to put the Qur'an down. I don't want to stop reading it even to eat or to sleep. When I read it, I feel connected to the rich history of those who were tested before me and who rose in status due to their patience in overcoming their trials.

It reminds me that I am not the only one who is being tested:

{Or do you think that you will enter paradise while such [trials] have not yet come to you as came to those who passed on before you? They were touched by poverty and hardship and were shaken until [even their] messenger and those who believed with him said: When will come the help of Allah? Verily, the help of Allah is near.}

(al-Baqarah 2:214)

We come from a history of individuals and nations who persevered, even through immense difficulties. Such is the nature of this ephemeral world: we will face all manner of difficulties. This is how Allah (swt) distinguishes those who are patient from those who lose hope.

For every moment of weakness, sadness, distress, and pain, it is only the Qur'an that can provide true healing. It was sent down by the Most Merciful to give us hope and faith in a time when most people look for remedies in things and places that provide only temporary numbness from their pain. No amount of physical or psychological intoxicants, though, can make you forget what is broken inside your soul.

{O mankind, there has to come to you instruction from your Lord and healing for what is in the breasts and guidance and mercy for the believers.}   *(Yoonus 10:57)*

November 12, 2013

I am astounded when people make excuses for those who support the killing of their brethren in Egypt and elsewhere. Many have tried to excuse their behaviour by saying they are brainwashed by the media or by their political or religious leaders. I don't believe in this brainwashing they speak of. I believe that Allah gave us enough intellect to distinguish between right and wrong.

{And Satan will say when the matter has been concluded: Indeed, Allah had promised you the promise of truth. And I promised you, but I betrayed you. But I had no authority over you except that I invited you, and you responded to me. So do not blame me; but blame yourselves. I cannot be called to your aid, nor can you be called to my aid. Indeed, I deny your association of me [with Allah] before. Indeed, for the wrongdoers is a painful punishment.}

(Ibrâheem 14:22)

No one is to blame for someone's misguidance except the person who is misguided. Even Satan and his agents will sell you out in the end. Satan whispers but you are the one who acts. Although the forces of media are strong, they are not stronger than the human mind, which should be able to listen, filter through the lies, and arrive at the truth. However, the mind has to be consciously employed to achieve this end.

I pray for the guidance of the people before they are brought to account in front of Allah over what their hearts believed, what their mouths said, and the immense bloodshed their complacency brought forth.

November 14, 2013

When the burden on my shoulders is heavy, I remember this verse:

{[Allah] will say: How long did you remain on earth in number of years?

They will say: We remained a day or part of a day; ask those who enumerate.

He will say: You stayed not but a little – if only you had known.}   *(al-Mu'minoon 23:112-114)*

Then I know that all I need to do is take one more step, pray one more prayer, live one more day. No pain lasts forever. What is on this earth will fade and what is with Allah will remain.[16]

It is just as Ibn Al-Qayyim has said, "O you who are patient! Bear a little more, just a little more remains."

November 15, 2013

When Amr was killed, I received messages from every inhabited continent on this earth, from people who were making *du'a* for him, for me, and for Ruqaya.

In the few days following his passing, my friends made *du'a* for him in the blessed Al-Aqsa Mosque in Palestine and his friend made *du'a* for him at the Prophet's Mosque in Madinah. At least twenty *'umrahs* were performed on his behalf; some were performed by people who had never even met us. His friend performed hajj on his behalf. Amr's friends recently launched a charity project in his name and they have already raised more than triple their monetary goal. There is more that I can't mention and I'm sure there is more that I don't know about, but I do know that his passing changed many lives – including mine.

I wonder, O Abu Ruqaya, what secret deed you had between you and Allah that He honoured you with such a death? Perhaps it was your habitual fasting, perhaps it was your night prayer, perhaps it was your relationship with the Qur'an, perhaps it was your love and mercy towards our child and me, or perhaps it was your respect for your parents.

Amr wasn't a renowned scholar or a well-known personality, but his deeds made him well known after he passed away.

Through all of this, I have learned that Allah (swt) is *al-Kareem*, the Most Generous. You may perform one tiny, seemingly insignificant good deed but because of your sincerity, Allah will multiply it manifold. Then, when you reach the Day of Reckoning, you may see that the deed you once thought was insignificant will be the means of you entering paradise.

Do not belittle any good act. You don't know just how generous your Lord can be. I ask *al-Kareem* to multiply our very few good deeds and help us enter the gates of paradise, where all our worries and fears will melt away.

November 17, 2013

Meet me by the edge of my dreams,
In the moments I drift into your realm.

Reach for me where you will find me –
Perhaps I may dream of you and your smile.

Find me amongst the souls that wander;
Call my name –
Perhaps I will hear your voice and come.

Perhaps time will not hurt as it does if your hand
    touches my forehead again and tells me:
      Nothing in this world is worth your tears.

November 18, 2013

My dear Ruqaya,

"Baba" is the sweetest word that has ever formed on your lips.

November 19, 2013

It is second nature for me to say *"alhamdu lillah"* when someone asks me how I'm doing. I rarely used to think about what that truly meant.

What it should mean is that I thank Allah for everything, every state of being. I thank Him for what I have and I thank Him for what I don't have. If He had given me everything I desired, perhaps it would have been a means for me to forget Him and go astray.

Now whenever I say *alhamdu lillah*, it's all-inclusive. It's a form of submission, an admission that I know nothing and He knows everything. It's an expression of trust and reliance on Him. I trust that He has given me exactly what I need to lead me back to Him.

Alhamdu lillah.

November 25, 2013

{From the earth We created you, and into it We will return you, and from it We will extract you another time.}

(Ṭâ Hâ 20:55)

Amr and I visited a beautiful little forest together in the summer of 2012. He fell in love with it, as he always did with nature. Thick forests are, of course, non-existent on the sand- and dust-laden shores of Alexandria. In this beautiful forest, Amr walked on the beaten path between the trees and stopped to touch their thick trunks, all the while praising Allah (swt) for the beauty of His creation.

I returned to this little forest today to see it slowly shedding its leaves in preparation for the cold winter. The contrast between the thriving greenery of the summer forest and the cold, sparse emptiness of the winter forest was striking.

It made me contemplate the fragility of life: how something or someone that seems so strong can perish from this earth in a moment simply by the will of Allah.

We are on this earth for a mere season and, like the leaves in this forest, we will also change and fall to the ground at our appointed time. *Subhan Allah.*

May Allah (swt) bless you with multitudes of forests and gardens, dear Amr: more beautiful and lasting than any on this earth.

May Allah (swt) guide our lives' seasons to be ones of exceptional obedience to Him; may He cause our passing to be as peaceful as a falling leaf; may He allow our souls to ascend to the heavens in peace; and may He resurrect us as strong, bright, and beautiful believers once again.

December 1, 2013

When this world became tight for you and when your path became too narrow, Allah (swt) set you free. So roam the heavens, my Amr, and laugh that contagious laughter of yours. You know better than I that you will never be a caged bird again.

December 3, 2013

Allah (swt) promises us that no suffering will be forgotten, that no good deed will be lost, and that an eternal home awaits those who are steadfast:

{And their Lord responded to them: Never will I allow to be lost the work of [any] worker among you, whether male or female; you are of one another. So those who emigrated or were evicted from their homes or were harmed in My cause or fought or were killed – I will surely remove from them their misdeeds, and I will surely admit them to gardens beneath which rivers flow as reward from Allah, and Allah has with Him the best reward.}   *(Âl-'Imrân 3:195)*

December 3, 2013

As I recall the beautiful friendships that have been a gift and blessing from Allah (swt) to support me through my difficulties, I remember this powerful hadith:

The Prophet (saws) said:

"Among Allah's servants are people who are neither prophets nor martyrs, but whom the prophets and martyrs will deem fortunate because of their high status with Allah. The Companions responded: O Messenger of Allah! Inform us of who they are.

He said: They are people who loved each other for Allah's sake, without being related to one another or being tied to one another by the exchange of wealth. By Allah, their faces will be luminous and they will be upon light. They will feel no fear when the people will be feeling fear and they will feel no grief when the people will be grieving. Then he read the verse:

{Behold! Verily on the friends of Allah there shall be no fear, nor shall they grieve.}   *(Yoonus 10:62)* "[17]

I have been blessed in my life to have the friendship of women who support and encourage every positive endeavour I undertake. They come to my aid whenever I ask for help and stand by my side even when I don't have the courage to ask. Our parents' mother tongues are not the same, we come from vastly different backgrounds, and our families' cultural practices could not be any more different yet we have found friendship based on the love of Allah (swt) and striving to better ourselves.

85

I am grateful for them every day. They lighten the darkness, they alleviate the sadness, and they walk with me on this road of healing. I pray that Allah (swt) alleviates their distress and fear on the Day of Judgment on account of joining hands with me for His sake.

December 4, 2013

No matter how severe your pain, rest assured that over time everyone will forget you. Just as the days that pass cause your body to age, just as assuredly as time moves forward and seasons change – rest assured that no one will remember your pain in a year or two.

Bide your time and remove your heart from the hands of people, then, and place it in the hands of Allah. Only there will you find true rest under the ever-watchful, ever-caring gaze of the One Who never forgets.

December 9, 2013

It was reported from 'Abdullah ibn Mas'ood (ra) that the Prophet (saws) said:

"No person suffers any anxiety or grief, and says:
O Allah, I am Your slave, son of Your slave, son of Your female slave, my forelock is in Your hand, Your command over me is forever executed, and Your decree over me is just. I ask You by every name belonging to You which You named Yourself with, or revealed in Your Book, or You taught to any of Your creation, or You have preserved in the knowledge of the unseen with You, that You make the Qur'an the life of my heart and the light of my breast, and a departure for my sorrow and a release for my anxiety – but (that) Allah will take away his sorrow and grief and give him joy in their stead."[18]

December 14, 2013

There is no better feeling than raising your hands to Allah and admitting your need to Him. Just simply saying, "I need You, Allah" is healing in and of itself. In that moment, you open your hands with palms facing towards the sky and let every worry and every stress float upwards, lightening your burdened hands.

{Is not He [best] who listens to the [soul] distressed when it calls on Him, and who relieves its suffering...?}

(an-Naml 27:62)

When I struggle to find the right words to say, or the right *du'a* to express my need, I just stop and say, "I need You, Allah."

I lay out all of my sorrows and pain and I hand them over to Him. He takes them from me and fills my hands with mercy and healing instead.

O Allah, become the ears with which I hear, the eyes with which I see, the hands with which I grasp, and the feet with which I walk.[19]

December 15, 2013

About two months ago I met a good friend of mine and we were walking by Lake Ontario with Ruqaya. As we were leaving each other's company, I told her, "If I had the choice to change what happened to Amr, I wouldn't." She told me that she was amazed at that statement and at my strength.

On the drive home, I reproached my soul for what I thought was a lie. I wished I had not said what I had said. Truthfully, my heart was aching for my husband and best friend and I would have done anything or given anything for him to return to me.

As time passed and Allah (swt) blessed me with a bit more understanding, I started to see the merit of that statement I had initially regretted saying. Now I can truly say that if I had the choice, I wouldn't change what happened to Amr. It's not because every day isn't a tremendous struggle and not because it isn't eating away at my heart whenever I see Ruqaya's doe eyes staring at a picture of her Baba. Rather, it is because wanting him back would mean that I trust my own judgment above Allah's wisdom and judgment. How could I say that it would be better if something different happened besides what Allah (swt) willed? I couldn't say that. I couldn't believe that.

I don't know why I said what I said then, but perhaps those words came directly from my heart so that Allah (swt) would guide me to reflect on them later. Even through the pain, I always believe that Allah has something better in mind for me: a better plan in this world and a better destination in the hereafter, *in sha'Allah*.

My Lord, I accept. I am satisfied with You as my Lord, with Islam as my faith, and with Muhammad (saws) as the final prophet.[20]

December 16, 2013

From the day I married Amr until the day he returned to his Lord, I never once had to set my alarm for the *fajr* prayer. Without fail, he would always be the one to wake me.

While we were in Egypt, the echoes of the *adhan* from the mosque near our home would wake him and he would make *wudoo* and shuffle down the stairs of our building to pray in congregation. He would wake me upon his return. It was the same while we were in Canada. Although he wasn't often able to pray *fajr* at the mosque, he would always be the one to set the alarm and get me up.

Once, in the sleeplessness and stress of having a newborn baby, we were so exhausted that we both slept through the alarm and missed the *fajr* prayer. That entire day Amr's face was dark with sadness, as though he had lost something incredibly valuable and dear to him.

Even though it was out of his hands, I understand now why it was so hated for him to lose a single prayer. Every prayer counts. Missing one means you've missed a chance at forgiveness from and closeness to your Lord.

On that most difficult day four months ago, he was killed right after performing the *'asr* prayer. He met his Lord just after he had been seeking nearness to Him.

May Allah (swt) keep you close and within His mercy, Amr, as you kept His remembrance close to your heart. May He honour you because of your respect of and adherence to the daily prayers and your love for the mosque.[21]

December 17, 2013

Sometimes I close my eyes and imagine a day, not too far away, when Allah (swt) will gather the souls of all the people who have ever walked this earth.

I imagine arriving at the pool of *al-Kawthar* and drinking from its water that will forever quench my thirst. I hope the water will be sweet; I hope it will quench the thirst in my throat as well as the thirst that is in my heart.

I imagine entering a place where there are things that no eyes have seen or ears have heard, a place no human mind can perceive. Some people long for the riches they'll find there or the rivers of milk and honey. Some people long for its beautiful homes and lush gardens. I do, too.

What I long for the most, though, is peace: a quiet serenity that no material possession can purchase. I want every worry and detail of the world to fade into the distance. I want it to be as though it were a faint dream that I don't remember when I wake.

I want to meet my Lord with love and certainty and submission overflowing from my heart, and simply say:

My Lord, You called me, so I came.

December 19, 2013

I spoke to my mother on the phone a few days after Amr left this world. I told her, "I wish I could just die, too." As much as I had tried to be patient and to bear it, it hurt more than anything I had ever felt and those words just came out.

For a long time I replayed that statement in my mind and felt a looming sense of guilt over what I had said. I told myself that I wasn't patient enough and that I had failed the test that Allah (swt) had given me.

Then a friend of mine reminded me of the verse referring to the story of Maryam:

{And the pains of childbirth drove her to the trunk of a palm tree. She said: Oh, I wish I had died before this and was in oblivion, forgotten.} *(Maryam 19:23)*

Allah didn't respond to her cries by harshly saying, "Do not wish for death!" or "Be more patient!" Rather, it was said to her out of a great and wonderful mercy:

{...Do not grieve; your Lord has provided beneath you a stream.
And shake toward you the trunk of the palm tree; it will drop upon you ripe, fresh dates.
So eat and drink and be contented...} *(Maryam 19:24-26)*

How merciful Allah is to have shown us such a human and authentic example of a woman who was in so much pain that she uttered her wish for death. This was not just any woman: it was Maryam (as), the best and most righteous of all the believing women. He then demonstrates to us how He responded with assurance, mercy, and love:

{Do not grieve.}

Allah (swt) created us and understands that we have great weaknesses and that we are flawed and imperfect. Even the greatest men and women were human; they grieved just as we do. They did and said things they regretted in times of pain.

Know that even if you say or do something you regret, Allah (swt) is the Forgiving. As long as you're alive, you still have the chance to redeem yourself. You still have the chance to reclaim the patience and constancy that you thought were lost to you.

Allah wishes ease for us. He wishes to extend His love and mercy to us. He wishes to comfort us in our times of pain and sorrow. Always remember His merciful response:

{Do not grieve.}

That mercy is for you and me, too.

December 20, 2013

Ruqaya and I were at a friend's house today. My friend's husband's name is Amr. At one point, my friend wanted to ask her husband something and he was in another room, so she called out to him, "Amr?"

Ruqaya froze for a few seconds. She dropped the toy that was in her hand and walked to the doorway of the other room, carefully peering in to see who was there. She stared at the *other* Amr for a while, saw that it wasn't *her* Amr, and came back to play.

I didn't realize that she would remember Amr. I thought her memory would have been wiped clean of her father by now since she was only nine months old when he was killed. There was still a glimmer of some distant memory there, however: a single moment of recollection behind her eyes...

My heart hurts when I see other children interacting with their fathers. Ruqaya will never sit on Amr's shoulders, be chased by him around a park, or collapse into a fit of giggles when he tickles her. She'll have me, but I'm not *him*.

I always come back to this verse, which gives me a sense of Allah's great justice:

{And whoever kills a believer intentionally, his recompense is hell to abide therein, and the wrath and the curse of Allah are upon him, and a great punishment is prepared for him...}
(an-Nisâ 4:93)

Every day as I hold Ruqaya's hand and walk forward in life, I can't help but look toward the place her father would have occupied had these criminals not extinguished his life. I can't help but notice that no matter what I do, one of her hands is empty.

I pray that those guilty of killing our beloved Amr are met with Allah's punishment, at which point they will truly understand what they have done. That day, they will understand whose hands they have taken out of my daughter's hands.

December 22, 2013

When I was pregnant with "Bilal," Amr told me that he actually wanted the baby to be a girl who would look just like her mom. I couldn't quite picture myself with a little girl. I wasn't a fan of all the potential frilly dresses, princess stories, and hair bows. It scared me. I told Amr I wanted a boy who would look just like him.

When Ruqaya was born, she was a girl who looked just like Amr (and she still looks like him). She was a strange combination of what we both wanted.

I have never been more grateful for Ruqaya than I have throughout the past four months and ten days of my *'iddah*. She kept me smiling and playing when I could have spun into an irreversible depression. She gave me hope for the future when I could have succumbed to a dark mess of hopelessness. She held my hand and kept my head above water when I could have drowned in my own sorrow.

Allah (swt) gives us what He wishes. He gives us what He knows we will need. He knew I would need this little girl and her smiles and her gentleness. He knew I would need her to need me so that I could get up in the morning and do what needed to be done.

It was never Bilal who I needed. It was Ruqaya.

For all those months of pregnancy, I didn't know who was in my womb. But He knew and He planned.[22] And Allah is the best of planners.

Alhamdu lillah.

December 24, 2013

My dear Ruqaya,

I see your wide eyes that soak in your surroundings and those ears that pick up words and make them form on your little lips as though you had been studying them for months. I can see my own reflection in your stare. The depth of emotion and thought that are developing in you astound me daily.

I wonder who you will be, whose hearts you will touch (and perhaps whose hearts you will break). I hope you lift and touch more hearts than you break. I feel that you will, because you are my daughter and you are your father's daughter. He was a heart-mender, a kind soul – and you are like him in a way. Your face is peaceful and expressionless as you sleep, your eyelashes curl up sweetly, and your closed lips look as though you are keeping a delicious secret: all like your father.

You are stubborn like me, though. You do not cease to try at something or to pull at my leg until you've gotten what you came for or until you've succeeded in your goal. You will knock on the door not until you become tired but until it is opened for you. Be stubborn, little one. Do not cease to try to be better and do better and achieve better, even if those around you attempt to pull you down. You are my daughter. And I will never cease trying to make you better until I am buried in the earth.

You are both of us, my cherub. You have the sweet but fiery temperament of your father. You have his humour and mischievous eyes. You have my stubbornness. You have my depth of love.

You are also different. Your soul is unique and although I do not know who you will be or what you will do, I have faith and hope in you. Not the kind of hope where I yearn for you to be a doctor or business owner – although you can be, if you wish.

My hope is that you will leave the world better than you found it. This is your purpose. This is who you were meant to be. This is who we are all meant to be.

Love,
Mama

December 25, 2013

Four months and ten days have passed. My mourning period is over. I must hold my head and heart up and return to some semblance of normalcy.

But the truth is, it still feels like you just left me yesterday.

Love, Unraveling

"You will be with the ones whom you love."

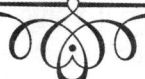

The gold moon

A few days after Amr passed away, his cousin had a dream of a full moon. It was a beautiful golden colour and there was a gold chain wrapped around its outer edge. She said the moon was that colour because of Amr.

Since I was a child, I have always loved the moon. Perhaps my love comes from the serenity and calmness of its light or the strange shadows on the bright full moon.

The moon is quieter and less dramatic than the sun. It's a metaphor for finding light in the darkness.

Before they even taught me how to pray, my parents taught me to look at the moon and say to it, "My Lord and your Lord is Allah," teaching me to consciously connect everything back to the Creator.

On my way back to Toronto from Egypt, my family picked me up at the airport. It was almost midnight. I strapped Ruqaya into her car seat and sat next to her in silence, wondering how it would be to go "home" without the second half of my heart with me. And as I looked out of the window, there it was as though waiting: the moon, a deep resounding golden colour as I have never seen it before.

It was not the full moon, only half.

It was the same moon from the dream. What strange peace it brought to my heart at that moment and how thankful I was that Allah was comforting me.

Accepting what comes

The funny thing is, I didn't really want to meet Amr and he really didn't want to meet me. My uncle set us up and I agreed to that first meeting just because I was too embarrassed to refuse his kind gesture. Amr was too embarrassed to reject him because he respected my uncle. They were neighbours and Amr didn't want to cause offense.

It was written long before either of us ever existed that we would meet (albeit reluctantly). It was that one meeting that clinched our interest in one another. As they say, the rest is history!

I wonder sometimes how much we fight against the will of Allah (swt), against fate, against what was written for us. Why can't we face each day just thinking: *I will accept what comes?*

The people who come into your path were meant to be there. If they leave or are taken, they were meant to leave you: all for a purpose.

When I look back at that time, Allah (swt) was giving me the most beautiful gift of Amr. Since He will never cease to be *al-Wahhab,* the Giver of gifts, who is to say that Amr's departure isn't also a beautiful gift, in a way? A gift wrapped in hardship but a gift nonetheless.

This is my hope, my dream, my longing – that a day will come when I will see the fruits of these beautiful and difficult gifts and that the love I have lost will be restored.

"When Allah tests you, it is never to destroy you. When He removes something in your possession, it is only in order to empty your hands for an even greater gift."

(Ibn al-Qayyim)

Holding back love

During all the evident happiness of getting engaged and preparing for our life together, Amr never told me he loved me. The words never escaped his lips. He waited to share these words with me once we were married several months later.

We never went out without a proper chaperone and even after we were engaged, our conversations were always within earshot of our families. None of this diminished our happiness. Our happiness was actually enhanced by this.

From the first time I met him, Amr struck me as a man with an integrity that is not easily matched. He understood the value of love and the value of maintaining modesty, even in a relationship that would end up being the closest relationship of our lives. He respected me enough to hold off on the things he may have really wanted to say. His desire to maintain his obedience to Allah was greater.

I am grateful that Amr never told me he loved me until our wedding day. He taught me that love – real, merciful, lasting love – is sacred. That which is given from your heart is the most valuable gift you can give someone. It's only fitting that you give your love carefully, at the right time, in the right place, and in a way that is pleasing to your Lord.

I am grateful for Amr every day.

Alhamdu lillah.

Forgiveness and gratitude

Amr taught me the true meaning of forgiveness and gratitude.

If we had an argument, we would never go to sleep angry or upset with one another. Without fail, one of us would always take the other's hand, relent, and apologize. It was never about who was right and who was wrong. Rather, it was about maintaining mutual love and respect for one another and recognizing that there were few things worth getting in the way of our relationship.

Every time I cooked a meal for him, helped him with a job application, or did him any favour, no matter how small, he would thank me. He was grateful to me for being his partner, for walking forward in life with him through the good and bad. That gratitude between us became the basis of our relationship.

This reminds me of a beautiful statement by Ibn al-Qayyim (ra):

Allah loves His attributes and characteristics, and He loves to see the effects of His attributes on His slaves. As He is beautiful, so He loves beauty; as He is all-forgiving, He loves forgiveness; as He is generous, He loves generosity; as He is all-knowing, he loves the people of knowledge; as He is strong and powerful, so a strong believer is more beloved to Him than a weaker one; as He is *as-Saboor* (the Patient), so He loves those who have patience; as He is *ash-Shukoor* (the Appreciative), so He loves those who give thanks.

As He loves those who have His characteristics, so He is with them, and this is a special and unique type of companionship.

Every day that passes is another day I gain appreciation for the kind of man Amr was. With me he always chose forgiveness over ego, generosity over miserliness, gratitude over thanklessness, and kindness over harshness. These qualities made him beloved to me and I hope that these qualities made him beloved to Allah.

I pray that I am also able to be patient, forgiving, grateful, and generous so that Allah (swt) may be all of those things towards me.

The best of men

This memory always makes me smile...

One Egyptian winter night before *'isha* prayer, I had a serious ice cream craving. Since Amr was going out to pray at the mosque right near our home, I asked him to buy me some. He agreed.

Just as the *'isha* prayer ended, a thunderstorm began – and Egyptian winter thunderstorms can be quite treacherous. Since Amr had left home in just flip-flops and a *galabiyah* (without an umbrella), I thought for sure he'd just run home and take cover. Twenty minutes later, he showed up bearing said ice cream for me. He was soaked from head to toe, laughing.

The Messenger of Allah (saws) said:

"The believers who show the most perfect faith are those who have the best behaviour, and the best of you are those who are the best to their wives."[23]

I know Amr was from the best of men because he was always the best to me. He knew that the simplest acts of love, kindness, and sacrifice were the best way to bring hearts together.

May Allah (swt) – the Merciful, the Loving – continuously honour him and raise his rank for the mercy and love he gave us without restraint.

Winter boots

A few months after we arrived in Toronto, the city was hit by a huge snowstorm. It was Amr's first time seeing snow and he took pleasure in throwing snowballs at me and making snow angels. It was also his first time experiencing walking on treacherously slippery and unsalted icy sidewalks. He bought a pair of sturdy boots to battle his first Canadian winter.

For several months after he passed away, the boots sat untouched in my closet. After hearing about the immense difficulties Syrian refugees overseas were encountering in the bitter cold, however, I decided to send the nearly-new boots there as a donation.

Part of me wanted the boots to stay in my closet forever to remind me of him. But I thought to myself: *perhaps this small act of kindness will reach someone far away and he will raise his hands and make* du'a *for the owner of these boots. Perhaps it will be counted among Amr's good deeds because something that belonged to him is bringing benefit to another human being.*

One *du'a* for him and one more good deed for him are so much dearer to me than holding onto what he owned.

Maybe when Amr stands before Allah (swt) on the Day of Judgment and sees his good deeds, he will wonder why he does not recognize some of them and he will be told: *The people who loved you did these deeds on your behalf.* How beautiful that would be and how honoured I would be to bring him one more moment of happiness! Although he's no longer with me, I still yearn to give him gifts. I pray that Allah (swt) allows this gift to reach his scale of good deeds.

I know that in the grand scheme of things, this is such an insignificant act and I do not even know who these boots will reach. However, I do know that Allah (swt) is *al-Kareem*, the Most Generous. He is capable of multiplying our smallest deeds and making them weigh heavily on our scales.

You don't own whatever is still in your hands. You only own the reward for that which you have given away for His sake. If you love someone, give him a gift that will weigh heavily on his scales.

May Allah (swt) accept and multiply our little actions and may He grant us a love that is greater than any worldly love: His love.

Living with the Qur'an

Amr was killed eight days after Eid ul-Fiṭr. That Ramadan, he finished reading the Qur'an three times: one full reading every ten days. For reasons unknown to me, he decided to set aside more time than usual to make sure he read as much Qur'an as possible.

Prophet Muhammad (saws) said:

"Whoever reads a letter from the Book of Allah, he will have a reward, and this reward will be multiplied by ten. I am not saying that *alif, lam, meem* is a letter; rather, I am saying that *alif* is a letter, *lam* is a letter, and *meem* is a letter."[24]

The Qur'an contains 323,671 letters. If every letter counts for ten rewards and Amr finished it three times, that means 9,710,130 rewards were recorded for him, *in sha' Allah,* multiplied manifold.

It was a beautiful end to a beautiful life.

Even though I sometimes try to comfort myself by meticulously counting and calculating Amr's deeds, I know that Allah's generosity knows no bounds and He has the power to multiply and increase so much more than I can calculate.

May Allah (swt) continuously increase my love's status for every letter of the Qur'an that he recited and memorized. May He accept from us the deeds that we think are small and multiply them manifold. May we be given the honour of having the Qur'an intercede for us. *Ameen.*

Still alive

Aside from some blood on his face, Amr's body in the hospital morgue was peaceful and silent as though he were only asleep.

I wished he really were only asleep, that I would hear his alarm soon, and that he would get up groggily asking, "What time is it?" Allah has decreed that death is final, though. No one comes back to this world once he leaves.

A man whose job it was to wash the bodies of the deceased before placing them in their shrouds washed Amr's body. He attended the funeral prayer and approached Amr's father saying, "Your son was different from most other people whose bodies I have washed. He must have had some special good deed he used to do."

He made this statement because Amr looked peaceful and the colour of his skin didn't change from Friday afternoon when he was killed until Saturday afternoon when he was buried. The man said that most bodies quickly become discoloured with bruise-like splotches on their skin.

He looked as though he were still alive.

Someone recently told me of a dream she had of Amr. He was leaning on the trunk of a towering tree so large that it extended far beyond what her eyes could see. He said to her, "We are not dead; we are alive." She said she had to tell me right away as she knew the message was meant for me.

I trust that Amr is alive and with Allah (swt), living the life of eternity that we were created to live. We were never meant to build a lasting home here. It makes me wonder how satisfied I was with this world and its details before Amr was taken. I was not evil but I was comfortable and complacent.

I am no longer comfortable here. My heart is not alive here.

Amr met the angel of death with a dignity that I can only hope for. He is the one living; I am the one who still has to emerge from the "death" of this world into the life of the hereafter.

We have only one soul, one chance. We spend some days or years on this earth before our fates will be sealed. Many of us will wish we could come back for another chance at life, but it will be too late. I pray that we leave this world with ease, that Allah (swt) covers us with His mercy which envelops all things, and that we do not bite down on our hands in regret for neglecting to accept the truth.[25]

{If you could but see when they are made to stand before the fire and will say: Oh, would that we could be returned [to life on earth] and not deny the signs of our Lord and be among the believers.} *(al-An'ām 6:27)*

Meeting Amr in my dreams

I dreamt of Amr. He was standing in a place that housed expensive things, as though it were a store of valuable jewels. I entered and he hugged me for a long time. After the hug, I saw that there were two large guards standing at the entrance of that place. They made me leave and they made Amr stay. Shortly thereafter, I woke up.

{It is Allah Who takes away the souls at the time of their death, and those that die not during their sleep. He keeps those [souls] for which He has ordained death and sends the rest for a term appointed. Verily, in this are signs for a people who think deeply.}   *(az-Zumar 39:42)*

The morning after that dream, the long hug we shared lingered in my every sense, as though he had really hugged me. In His wisdom, however, Allah (swt) sent my soul back to my body and gave me another chance at life, another day to try to attain His pleasure. I know Amr had to stay where he was, but we will all eventually return to the One Who created us. This is not our home. This is not our destiny. Our existence in this world is like a single moment of rest under the shade of a tree. Soon we will get up and continue our journey into the hereafter.

It was a strange dream, a beautiful dream.

What else is paradise except a place like I saw: a place that houses expensive things created for the believers by Allah (swt)? What greater price can one pay to receive those things than his or her life?

Our existence is, in a sense, merely an exchange of goods. We are seeking to purchase the best and most lasting thing, which is paradise, but we have to pay the price for it. We have to live, not for the benefit of our current selves in a world that values selfish desires, but for our future selves: our selves that need, more than anything else, to be given a home in paradise, by the mercy of Allah (swt).

The Prophet (saws) said:

"…Each one of us goes forth in the morning as a vendor for his soul. He either achieves its emancipation or brings it to perdition."[26]

Amr's grave

Amr and I spent hours, days, and months working on our apartment in Egypt so it would be in perfect condition when we moved in (to be honest, he actually did most of the work). According to Egyptian tradition, every single thing in our apartment had to be new and spotless. We renovated, painted, and bought new furniture. For weeks, Amr would leave the pharmacy once his shift was over and go to our apartment to diligently keep track of the renovations.

We lived there for only a year before moving to Canada. As we were leaving, we covered all the furniture, disconnected the appliances, and locked the door tightly. We wanted to protect what was inside.

No one could bear to go back to that apartment after Amr was killed. I haven't seen my "treasured" things since then.

Our human culture places immense value on the physical spaces we occupy. We aim for perfection in our homes. We strive to have every piece of furniture match every rug and every rug match every ornament. Yet soon all of it will fade into nothingness.

When we die, we won't care that our apartments and houses and mansions were beautiful. The only place that will occupy our thoughts is the small compartment that will be our grave and whether we will have a door to paradise or a door to hell swung open for us.

I can't bear to go see the things that were once beloved to me. I can't gather the courage to open the door and find the things we had arranged just so. I can't understand the purpose of those things anymore now that my love has gone.

117

I often wonder whether I have put the same effort into adorning my house in paradise as I put into perfecting the physical space we lived in for such a short time. I know now that there is no home here. Every moment we spend working towards permanency in this place instead of working towards our salvation will be a moment we regret.

I don't know what is left in this world for me. I don't yet know what paths I will walk or to what places I will be taken.

I do know, though, that walking the quiet, dusty path towards Amr's grave and sitting there for some moments would surely give me more contentment than sitting on the couch we picked out together.

May Allah take me there again one day.

Wanderer

Where is home?

People say home is where the heart is. They say home is not defined by the space between four walls of a house. Rather, home is defined by love, attachment, and where you yearn to be.

I had a home once. I remember Amr taking my hand and saying, "You are my home." I was his home on this earth and he was mine. Now that he's gone from this world, I often feel like a wanderer with no roots, no sense of belonging. Nowhere feels right or cozy or warm. Nowhere is *home* anymore.

What is the remedy for a homeless heart except to travel toward the true Home? To seek refuge and shelter from this season's dark and cold elements with Allah, *as-Samad*: the Eternal Refuge. Everything changes but Him. Every shelter is torn down but His.

Home is where the father and mother of humanity first lived. It's where they were first happy together. Home is a place of limitless beauty outside the shackles of time and space.

It's not where you go once your shift is over. It's not where you eat your meals or change your clothes. That "home" is just a temporary space you are occupying for some moments.

Yes, Home is where the heart is.

Perhaps my question should have never been, "Where is home?" I know Home is paradise.

The question should be, "Where is my heart?" It's either longing for the true Home or longing for someplace else.

From his hand to mine

During my first Ramadan with Amr, we went to *taraweeh* prayer at the largest congregation in Alexandria. Thousands of people gathered to pray in the open air by the sea. They blocked traffic, lining every narrow street and filling every empty lot.

When the prayer was over, some young men were walking around with donation boxes, collecting money for the victims of a severe famine in Somalia. I rifled through my purse to get some of my money together, handed it to Amr, and he gave it to one of the men collecting donations.

My last Ramadan with Amr, we prayed *taraweeh* at a local mosque in Alexandria. As we were heading home, we saw an elderly woman sitting on the side of the road asking passersby for money. He took a bill out of his wallet, put it in my hand, and asked me to go give it to her. I did and she made *du'a* for us.

It was one of the last things we did together.

Charity from my hand to his, from his hand to mine. That's how it was between us and that's how it is with love, at least when you don't love selfishly and when you understand that there is a greater purpose to love and to life. You give together, you pray together, you become better together.

Both my first and last Ramadan experiences with Amr were punctuated by these events and they have stayed with me. The image of Amr emerging from the men's side of the mosque with a wet beard has also remained. He never told me why he cried in those final prayers and I didn't ask.

One of the many things Amr taught me was the importance of giving: not just giving money to those in need, but giving of yourself to your family, friends, and community. I mean the kind of charity that is to be a positive force on this earth, to radiate goodness and fairness wherever you go and to give from what is most personally yours: your heart, your smile, your good words.

We don't really understand what charity means. It doesn't mean that the person giving is rich or noble or exceptionally philanthropic. Rather, those who continuously give are actually those who see themselves as the ones in need.

They need Allah's mercy, His forgiveness. They need to alleviate the distress of others so that Allah (swt) can alleviate their distress on the Day of Judgment. I think Amr realized how much we were in need of this, so he endeavoured to always give to me, our daughter, his friends, and his community. He never stopped giving until the day he returned to Allah.

He never stopped giving because he knew that he needed Allah to give him something greater. I pray that he has received something much, much greater than what he gave away.

Continuous charity

I recently received several pictures of a well built in Amr's name in an area of Pakistan where most families live far below the poverty line. The inhabitants of the area were forced to walk long distances to find clean water to drink, perform *wudoo*, and use for their daily needs.

The people responsible for raising the funds for this well have never met Amr or me. They weren't from the same country and we didn't have any shared networks or friends. They raised funds in Amr's name after hearing his story and now a small village has easy access to clean water because of the efforts of these individuals.

This reminds me of this beautiful hadith in which Allah's Messenger (saws) said:

"If Allah loves someone He calls (Angel) Jibreel and says: I love so-and-so, so you love him.
Jibreel loves him and calls the other angels in Heaven to love that person. They love him, then his love is made upon earth, and he becomes loved…"[27]

Amr lived his life in the framework of worshiping Allah and continuously serving others. He hoped for rewards from Allah and feared that if he should fall off this path of worship and service, he would incur Allah's displeasure. I hope that because of this, Allah (swt) has blessed him with the love of righteous people and the well as a source of continuous charity.

May Allah (swt) allow every drop of water that benefits the people, the animals, and the vegetation to be an addition to Amr's scale of good deeds. I pray that in his meeting with Allah (swt) on the Final Day, Amr will be surprised at these beautiful deeds that have accumulated for him.

Alhamdu lillah.

The bribe

Amr was in the habit of going out with his friends once a week. They did whatever guys do when they meet up: eat, talk politics, go bowling, and generally make a lot of noise.

Every week when he came home, he would bring me something: chocolate, ice cream, a fresh fruit drink from our favourite drink stand. He humorously joked with his friends that it was a "bribe" he had to pay his wife so she would allow him to hang out with his friends. Everyone knew that wasn't the case. It was just the immense goodness and love within him searching for different ways to express itself.

The gifts he brought home weren't significant and he didn't spend a lot of money on them. That was never the point. The point was that he knew the *sunnah* of gift-giving.

The Prophet (saws) said:

"Give gifts to one another and this will make you love each other."[28]

People seem to think that love is borne out of grand gestures and perfectly-phrased poetic declarations when in reality it is the little gifts that make love last: a regular smile, a kind word of encouragement, and yes – a chocolate bar. When you give gifts often, you are telling the person you love: *My love is constant. I do not forget you, even when we are apart.*

Above all, Allah (swt) is *al-Wahhab*: the Giver of gifts. He fills every single day of our lives with big and little gifts waiting to be unwrapped. His love is constant and He does not forget us, although sometimes we forget Him.

I often invoke Allah (swt) by His name, *al-Wahhab*. Knowing that He is constantly giving gifts to His servants makes me hopeful that my hands will always be full of gifts from Him.

There's only one way for me to reciprocate Amr's gifts to me now. I do not forget him, even when we are apart.

O Allah! I have entrusted to You the care of Amr, my most beloved gift. Have mercy on him, forgive him, and grant him Your love.

Equilibrium in faith

For many years in Egypt, Amr attended every one of the five prayers in congregation, regardless of where he was. It wasn't difficult considering there is a mosque on almost every street corner.

However, when we came to Canada he could no longer do that. We neither lived within walking distance of any mosques nor did we have a car. Something beautiful that he had been doing for so long was now out of his reach. It affected him in many ways and I could see the silent sadness reflected in his demeanor.

He didn't let himself stagnate, though. He began setting his alarm regularly and waking up before *fajr*. Then he stood and prayed the *tahajjud* prayer, reading the revelation of Allah alone in the dark until the time of the *fajr* prayer came.

Before this, I never knew Amr as an avid night-worshiper. He would wake up for *tahajjud* on occasion but not regularly. In establishing this new habit, he taught me something important about achieving equilibrium in faith and in life.

When we have circumstances that make it difficult to practice one recommended element of faith, we do not give up on faith altogether nor do we let a setback push us and keep us down. We revisit and reevaluate. Then we come to an understanding of what we can do to lift ourselves up again.

Believers never stagnate. They do not allow circumstances of life to control and dictate how they will live and worship. Amr wasn't physically able to pray in the mosque as often as he would've liked, so he found something else that would allow him to maintain the strength of his faith.

{O you who have believed, respond to Allah and to the Messenger when he calls you to that which gives you life. And know that Allah intervenes between a man and his heart and that to Him you will be gathered.} *(al-Anfâl 8:24)*

Worshiping Allah (swt) gave Amr life. It gave him the strength and conviction to live on the path of truth and to die on the path of truth.

One of the most recited *du'a*s of the Prophet (saws) was:

"O You Who changes the hearts, make my heart firm on Your religion.

When he was asked by his Companions about the meaning of this *du'a*, the Prophet (saws) said:

The hearts are between two of Allah's fingers. He changes them (as He wills)."[29]

Your heart is never traveling on one path, at one speed, unaffected by its surroundings. It is soft, malleable, ever-changing. It has its ups and downs, its facets of brightness and its shades of darkness. If left alone without worship or faith or striving, the heart will slowly rust and become unrecognizable. The believers are never stagnant. They are always seeking balance and equilibrium.

They are always searching for that which will give their hearts life.

Moving on

Losing you is like waking up to a world that has lost its sun. How is it that the world expects me to *move on* when losing you is like losing water in the heat of the desert?

Perhaps they have not felt the coolness of love as it is gulped in desperation by those with hearts as parched and aching as mine had been. Perhaps they do not understand the meaning of losing you, for you are not the only one lost, my love. I now wander from day to day having lost sight of you, having seen you cold, having seen things no woman can bear to see.

Yet I bear it because my child needs the sun to grow and play. I have lost you, my beautiful, radiant friend, so I take your place and shine so that she may one day know a love as bright as I have known.

This is how I choose to *move on*.

Scent

A bottle of Amr's perfume sits on the shelf in my closet. I brought it home with me along with a few other things that belonged to him. I had to leave most of his things behind but I took the bottle to remember his smell, to remember that everything I had was real, that he was real – that he is *still* real, in another place.

The sense of smell is powerful. It evokes memories and thoughts from times that have long since passed. It transports us to moments we thought were forgotten.

The martyr will be resurrected with his wounds smelling of musk,[30] while the fasting person's breath is sweeter than musk in the sight of Allah.[31] Amr was both of those things, by the permission and acceptance of Allah (swt). Since the day I met him, he fasted every Monday and Thursday[32] and the three middle days of the month,[33] without fail, unless he was sick or traveling. I fasted with him sporadically but I would become easily fatigued and lose motivation.

He, however, remained consistent and that is what is beloved to Allah (swt): to remain consistent in a deed, regardless of how minor it may seem.[34]

Allah (swt) remembers those who have sacrificed their comfort and lives by raising them above all others through a beautiful scent that will emanate from them. They will be recognized, envied, elevated. Their faces will be bright on a day when many faces will be darkened. Such is the reward for those who sacrifice their time and effort in pursuit of that which is loved by Him.

It's strange to think of this bottle of perfume that I have held onto so dearly, carrying it with me across oceans and periodically spraying it into the air to remember his scent. I am only human and I keep it to remind myself of a love that has evaded me, for a time. But it will perish as all else does. What is with Allah in deeds is the only thing of ours that will remain.

The ground that mourns

Somewhere in your hometown, a nondescript piece of asphalt is permanently stained with your blood: your precious, fragrant, expensive blood. I wonder – did the ground mourn as I do, having felt the remainder of your life seeping from your body? Did it curse your killer and promise to be a witness for you in front of Allah, having absorbed your blood into itself? Did it seethe with anger?

Your blood, I'm sure, has been smeared by passing cars, dried by the heat of the Egyptian sun, washed away by the torrid rains of the Egyptian winter. To the naked eye, what remains of you is gone.

I pity him, the poor soul behind the gun who was the cause in removing your soul from our lives. He will answer to Allah, the Just, on the Day of Reckoning. The witnesses against him will be many.

Regardless of the seasons and the elements, regardless of the time that elapses or the memories that become blurred and faded, that piece of ground will always be stained with your blood.

Traveling

Your plane ticket was booked to come home with me in just two days. Our suitcases were mostly packed. Your dinner was ready for when you returned that afternoon.

But your ticket to your real home in the hereafter was already booked far before we knew one another. You didn't need your suitcases because you had packed your good deeds away in a place where they are never lost and with a Keeper who never forgets.

I pray you have arrived at your destination without delays or worries. I pray you are safe in the protection and company of your Lord.

Echoes of you

Sometimes stars in the sky appear to still be there, their light reaching our eyes even though they have long since died. For me, you are that distant star in the night sky.

The echoes of your existence are still rippling through my atmosphere, as though you haven't quite gone. Your smell still lingers in your clothes, your roughly-used *miswak* still waits to be used again, your pocket Qur'an still rests on my shelf.

The echoes of your voice are still ringing in my ears: your boisterous laughter and quiet, constant words of mercy, humour, and love.

Even your face is still here, buried in the features of our daughter. Her downturned lips and arched eyebrows are yours. Her eyes, too, are yours as they look at me quizzically and mischievously. Her little voice bears the same bright tones of excitement your voice used to carry. When I ask her, "Where's Baba?" she replies, *"Jannah!"*

She still doesn't understand, but there are echoes of you in her.

Perhaps someday the light of that lone star will no longer be seen, perhaps the echoes will seem to be muted as they run their course, but you can never really be gone if you are alive with Allah.

And how, too, can you ever be gone when your light still reaches our hearts?

Growing young

I will never see your beard turn grey with age and wisdom, nor sweep away the stray white hairs that fall from it. I will never hold your aged hand and look into eyes wrinkled by time and laughter.

I will never grow old with you.

Now I hope for a place where I will grow *young* with you. It might take me just a few moments or many years to get there, but I am traveling to you.

I will discard the possessions and sins I don't need, the things that will add weight to my already burdened shoulders. I will never be able to sleep comfortably knowing that I need to continue traveling in the morning. No food will satisfy this hunger, no drink will quench this thirst.

The path to you is inhabited by thieves and covered in thorns and sinkholes, but I will gather my garments close to me and struggle not to fall until I am home.

The Prophet (saws) told us that Allah (swt) says:

"My faithful servant's reward from Me, if I have taken to Me his best friend from amongst the inhabitants of the world and he has then borne it patiently for My sake, shall be nothing less than paradise."[35]

My Lord, build for my family near You a home and a garden that will never fade nor rust nor age.

A seamless love

I was eight months pregnant and I was struggling to bend down and put on my own shoes. He knelt down, kissed my feet, put my shoes on for me and tied the laces. Then we left the house, all without him saying a word.

Amr.

He never said to me begrudgingly, "Remember how well I took care of you?" or "What will you give me in return for me doing this favour for you?"

That wouldn't be love. Love isn't empty grand gestures or keeping score on who wins which arguments. It's a quiet mercy, a steady stream of empathy and compassion. It's the ability to seamlessly be yourself while simultaneously being the person your partner needs you to be at any given moment.

Amr taught me that love is many things and, above all, that love and mercy is from Allah.

Prophet Muhammad (saws) said:

"Allah divided mercy into one hundred parts, out of which he retained ninety-nine parts with Him and sent down one part to earth. From this one part emanates all the compassion that all of creation exercises toward one another, so much so that an animal lifts its hoof above its young lest it should get hurt."[36]

Every ounce of overwhelming love and mercy that Amr had on me and our daughter is a manifestation of just *one* of the parts of mercy that Allah (swt) sent down to earth. How, then, could I ever despair of the mercy of Allah, who has kept with Himself ninety-nine?

Love, extending

My dear Ruqaya,

My baby daughter, when you point to your belly button and ask, with a grin on your face, "What's this?" My mouth says, "Belly button" but my heart says: *This is the mark on your body that connects me to you. It doesn't fade with age. It will always be there to remind you that my lifeblood is your lifeblood. You are a part of me; you grew with me, you ate with me, you cried with me. I felt you before I met you; I loved you before I knew you.*

When you look down at your belly button, know that although you are out in the world now, roaming, learning, laughing, and being, you are still from me, you are still within me. An umbilical cord no longer connects our bodies, but a love that cannot be cut will always connect our hearts.

{And We have enjoined upon man [care] for his parents. His mother carried him, [increasing her] in weakness upon weakness, and his weaning is in two years. Be grateful to Me and to your parents; to Me is the [final] destination.}

(Luqmân 31:14)

An eternal love

If you have loved, I mean *really* loved...

If you have taken hold of someone's hand, looked at him with understanding, then moved forward on your path saying: *Walk with me and I will walk with you; worship Allah with me; support me when I become fatigued and I will support you...*

When you have loved like that, whether romantically or otherwise, you can't believe that this world is all you get. You can't believe that the experience of love ends when your love goes to his temporary resting place. Love is something that lives even when you die. You do not part at death.

Love is eternal. Perhaps it becomes subdued. Perhaps it is sometimes muted by the shadows of stress and life. But it follows you. It staples itself to your garments and holds onto you even when you feel alone. True love: no, it never dies.

"You will be with the ones whom you love,"[37]

our beloved Prophet (saws) said. It's a fact. It's a promise. So love fully but love carefully as well.

Fighting a war within

Amr and I were married in a mosque in Alexandria, just steps from the Mediterranean Sea, called Masjid as-Salam: the Mosque of Peace. That is exactly what our marriage was: peaceful. It was like a breath of fresh, clean, seaside air amid the chaos and pollution of life.

Since Amr's departure, though, I have been at war. It's a war that no one can see or feel or touch. It's a war within my soul. I am fighting with patience, fighting to hold onto it, fighting to not succumb to asking one of the darkest questions of all: *Why me?*

Patience isn't always sweet. It's sometimes a bitter pill, a burden that makes its carrier hunch with exhaustion. Having one beautiful moment of true patience doesn't mean you are thereafter free from pain or that patience and trust in Allah become easy.

Despite all my efforts, despite believing that what Allah (swt) has planned for me is better than what I can ever dream for myself, sometimes I wish. Oh, how I wish. I wish so deeply, so intensely, so forcefully that I could breathe easily again for just one moment. I wish for that perfect seaside air of our wedding day. I wish to forget, for just a minute, the image of Amr's injured, lifeless body lying in the morgue.

But I can't forget.

Patience doesn't follow you. It isn't enslaved to you. If you turn your back on it for a moment, it will evade you. You cannot simply *be* patient. It's not a state of mind that can ever be fully achieved. It's a battle that must be fought daily.

I pray that in this struggle, I win against the darkness more often than I lose.

We belong to Allah

Around twenty minutes before Amr was shot and killed, I called him. I was worried but he quickly quelled my fears and said to me, "Don't worry. I'm on my way home now."

He was indeed on his way Home.

It wasn't the home that either of us had imagined, however. It wasn't the home where he would be sitting next to me, telling me about his day and having a meal with his family. It was his true Home: the home most of us forget about until we actually get there.

Verily to Allah we belong and to Him we shall return.

Amr returned to Allah: not to punish me or his family; not to cause us sleepless nights or sadness and anxiety; certainly not because some criminal "decided" to take his life.

He returned to Allah because Allah owns him and He decided it was time.

Allah (swt) continuously gives us gifts to bring us closer to Him and to help us thank Him. These gifts we have in our hands aren't for us to keep forever. We don't own them. Allah does. We just have them for a short period of time.

We attach our hearts to the physical gifts of which we are in possession. We love the gifts, we spoil the gifts, we hold tightly to the gifts. We ignore the Gift-giver, then when He takes the gift away we become angry and ungrateful as though we were the true owners of that something or that someone.

We own nothing. We don't even own ourselves.

Allah (swt) gave Amr to me as a gift for a time. By taking this gift away, Allah (swt) taught me more than I would have ever known had Amr still been with me. He taught me about pain, about courage, about sacrifice. He taught me to yearn for a true Home that is eternal. He taught me that no matter how much I dig my heels into this world, I will still return to Him at the time and place He wills.

Sometimes we need the gifts He gives us and sometimes we need Him to take them away. Perhaps only then will we understand our need and love for *the Source* of those gifts.

Never empty

Amr first held my hand the day we married. It was an extraordinary and beautiful feeling to hold my husband's hand for the first time.

He always held my hand as we crossed the overcrowded, perilous streets of Egypt half nervously walking, half running for our lives. He held my hand while I was in the throes of labour, his face weighed down with worry.

I remember my palms tingling, my fingers stretching and clenching themselves into a fist after he was killed. My hands were suddenly empty. My body was off balance as I tried to walk forward because I was used to leaning into the comfort and warmth of our clasped hands. I remember the pain that was within me somehow extending into my extremities.

There were times I felt as though nothing could replace the emptiness in my hands. There were times my hands felt heavy, plagued with a kind of paralysis, so burdened with the weight of pain that I didn't think I could do what needed to be done.

I did what needed to be done, however. I know now that it was because my hands were never really empty at all.

We raise our empty palms towards the sky when we make *du'a*. When we request something from Allah – forgiveness, mercy, healing, health – we often stare into our empty palms, memorizing the lines of age and creases of our skin. Isn't it befitting that we ask what we need of Allah (swt) with outstretched hands?

Without His blessings and sustenance, we would be destitute. Without His mercy, we would all be condemned to punishment for our misdeeds. Without His light, we would all be in perpetual darkness.

It is our bare, outstretched palms that help us understand that without Allah, we would have nothing and we would be nothing.

Prophet Muhammad (saws) said:

"Verily your Lord is generous and shy. If His servant raises his hands to Him (in supplication) He becomes shy to return them empty."[38]

I have lived this beautiful hadith. When my outstretched palms begged my Lord for relief and mercy and ease, He filled them. He filled them with my daughter's soft, mischievous, sticky toddler hands. He filled my life with ease of heart and the company of beautiful people.

Sometimes He didn't fill my hands with exactly what I had asked of Him but He filled them with what was better.

Amr's hands never returned to me. Perhaps one day they will, but as long as my palms are outstretched to my Creator, the last thing my hands are or ever will be is empty.

Your hands

I remember the first moments of holding your hand.
It felt instinctive for you to offer your hand to me,
and only natural for me to take it.

My heart was filled with a strange relief
as though all our shouldered worries
were as light as snowflakes brushed away by mittened hands,
as though my previous life had
disappeared into a past that I would never revisit.

It was your hands – your kind, unquestioning hands.
They made me want to tell you
that you had repaired something broken and weary,
sewed the ripped seams of my heart back together.
Your hands – holding me steady and keeping me balanced –
were a response to my silent prayers,
my quiet moments of gratitude and trust in Allah.

When I was waiting for them, waiting to be held and to hold,
I wondered if you'd ever come, and I doubted myself:
doubted that any other hand could fit into mine,
could feel as comfortable and smooth against my palms,
could store an exponential love between ten fingers,
    intertwined.

So we held on tight as though we were making up for lost time,
as though we would fall apart if our fingers weren't locked.
And I thought I would fall apart without your hands.

Then you let go.
Your hands fell to the pavement and I wasn't there.

143

My hands fell to my sides: hanging, waiting, grieving.
I wasn't there to hold you as your soul departed your body.
I couldn't reach you to help you, to carry you, to wrap you.

You were held by someone else,
ascending to where your Lord, Most High, was waiting
    for you.
I hope He filled your hands with rewards and coolness
    and peace.
I hope you rejoiced with what He gave you.

And the truth is I didn't fall apart without your hands.
I continued to walk, to pray, to breathe, to live,
even when I didn't want to.
Even when the earth seemed like a wasteland.
Even when the night was dark and perpetual.
Even when my utter brokenness was rattling inside me and
    the seams of my heart were almost undone.

I didn't fall apart.

But the weak, torn, imperfect, human seams around my
heart still hope that perhaps you are somewhere,
standing,
hands outstretched,
waiting for me.

Clothing

Right after Amr and I were married, the "Are you pregnant?" questions began flooding in from everyone we ran into: family, friends, distant acquaintances (Egyptians can be especially intrusive on this issue).

Once Amr and I were out together and he ran into an old friend who asked if I was pregnant. Amr stuck out his own stomach, patted it, and said, "We've actually decided that I will carry our first child." His friend laughed nervously and never asked that question again.

That became Amr's standard response.

When I remember that day (and every day with Amr) I am always reminded of what Allah (swt) says about spouses:

{...They are your garments and you are their garments...}
(al-Baqarah 2:187)

Out of love and respect for me, Amr chose to deflect the questions that he knew might bother me. He protected me like clothing protects us from the elements. He hid my faults. He shielded me. He was a source of ease and comfort for me.

Then he was suddenly gone and that garment fell away. I felt exposed and unprotected, like the whole world would be able to see right through me. My heart and my faults were out in the open for all to see. I felt like that for a long time.

Then I recently came upon this verse:

{O children of Adam, We have bestowed upon you clothing to conceal your private parts and as adornment. But the clothing of righteousness – that is best. That is from the signs of Allah that perhaps they will remember.}

(al-A'râf 7:26)

Allah (swt) says that the "clothing" of *taqwa* is the best of all clothing. The protection, closeness, and covering of a spouse may disintegrate over time or forcefully be pulled away from us, but we will always have access to the greatest garment of all: consciousness of Allah.

Striving to attain Allah's pleasure by simultaneously hoping in His mercy, fearing His punishment, and loving Him is the greatest protection and comfort that can ever be achieved.

He will hide our faults like clothing hides the blemishes on our skin. He will beautify us like beautiful clothing enhances our appearance. He will protect us like clothing protects us from the harsh elements.

I have spent so long yearning for my garment that was forcefully pulled from me. Now I know there's a better garment to replace the one I lost. I just have to consciously put it on.

Love, unraveling

A humanitarian aid worker was killed recently in Bashar al-Assad's Syrian prisons. I was blessed to be able to get in touch with his widow. She told me she saw a dream of her husband after his passing. In this dream she was inside her home looking out the window and he was outside looking in at her. She drew a heart on the fogged window and wrote in it: *"Jannah."* He smiled.

Those who do not know love think our love stories are over. Those who have not lived in the peace and tranquility of that miracle think our love stories end when our beloved ones are taken from us.

But as long as we have breath in our chests and tongues that remember Allah (swt), the names of our beloved will not leave our *du'as*. We will raise our children to uphold the strong legacies of their fathers and mothers. For as long as blood pumps through our bodies, we are running forward, climbing upward, fighting with our own souls so that we may enter paradise together, hand-in-hand with the ones who occupy our hearts.

Those who have killed think they've won, but instead their actions have yielded men and women who will not bow to anyone except Allah and who will do whatever it takes to meet Him and enter His mercy.

If this isn't our love stories still unraveling, still being told, still blooming more beautifully from one day to the next, then I am the one who doesn't know the meaning of love.

Voices of the Oppressed

"Beware of the supplication of the oppressed
for there is no barrier between it and Allah."

No good is wasted

The Arab Spring of January 2011 gave birth to the Egyptian revolution against Hosni Mubarak's thirty-year rule. That period of time brought out the best in some people and the worst in others. Hardened criminals were "mysteriously" set free from prisons and police officers who were loyal to the state vanished from the streets. No one was protecting the people.

Amr would take shifts with other men to guard the neighbourhood at night from the scores of looters and criminals who surfaced after the Egyptian police force decided to disappear. On one occasion, Amr and the other men captured a couple of people who were trying to burglarize and vandalize their area. I remember Amr retrieved a sword from one of them (yes, an actual sword). He kept it as a souvenir to show me.

Fast forward to today and it seems all that goodwill has died. People are regularly thrown into prison and murdered in the streets by the state regime that forced its way back into power. The murders and imprisonments have become so commonplace that it barely makes the news anymore.

Egypt is a textbook case of corruption. The oppressors are free and running the country; the good are silenced, either in prisons or in their graves.

I have heard some people say, "All our sacrifices went to waste. All the blood of all the martyrs went to waste."

To them I say what Yoosuf (as) said:

{...Indeed, he who fears Allah and is patient, then indeed, Allah does not allow to be lost the reward of those who do good.}   *(Yoosuf 12:90)*

In the sight of Allah (swt), no deed ever goes to waste.

As much as I miss Amr, I feel that Allah (swt) was merciful to him in that he was permitted to exit this world with honour. He shielded Amr from witnessing the mess that Egypt turned out to be. Perhaps it is fitting that those who were too soft-hearted for this pain were removed from the world before having their hearts broken.

This is other-worldly mercy.

Sacrifice

While I was living in Egypt in 2012, I took part in the first democratic elections following the January 2011 removal of Hosni Mubarak.

When I went to my assigned polling station, the line of women was outrageously long. I was pregnant at the time and couldn't bear to stand in the sun for two hours in order to vote. My mother-in-law was with me and spoke to one of the guards, who allowed me to proceed to the front of the line.

Needless to say, there was no voter apathy. Even I, as the "foreigner" that most people saw me to be, cared enough to take my tired, pregnant body to the polling station. The lines spilled onto the streets and had to be managed by soldiers.

At the time there was a sense of cautious hope for a better Egypt, perhaps an Egypt where my children would be proud to visit and live. Many things have changed since then, though.

After everything that has happened, after all the sacrifice and pain and loss, I wonder now to myself: would I be willing to give my life fighting for justice? Would I have the courage to stand up for what's right if the time came, regardless of the consequences?

This isn't a political question. This isn't even really about Egypt. This is just a question that I ask myself when I sometimes compare myself to Amr. He insisted on standing in solidarity with the oppressed and speaking in support of justice. He made the greatest sacrifice anyone could make.

My greatest fear is that if I were to be put in a similar situation, I wouldn't have that bravery or conviction to sacrifice everything for the truth. What is the meaning of life, then, if you don't live and die by the principles of truth and justice?

I ask Allah for strength so that I may be brave enough to be present in the struggles that truly matter and to fear no one but Him.

Voices of the oppressed

I miss Amr's voice: the way its tones filled every corner of the house and held me together when I was exhausted, the way it was a constant comfort in a fragile and inconstant world, the way it calmed me in times of stress.

His voice was silenced.

Millions of voices like his have been silenced. By the end of time, perhaps the number of voices that have been silenced will be far greater than any historian can count. However, the ultimate record of Allah is accurate; He will know their numbers.

They have been silenced by threats, by being witness to unspeakable pain, by being imprisoned. Many have been silenced by simply being wiped off the face of the earth.

On the Day of Reckoning, their voices will be returned to them. They will have a platform. They will be asked: *For what crimes were you killed?* and then they will speak with absolute clarity. Being given permission to speak that day is truly a great honour.

Those who did the silencing – the ones who held their guns and fired at will, the ones who harassed, demonized, and abused; the ones who lied to legitimize murder and war – they will be the ones who are silenced.

{That day, We will seal over their mouths, and their hands will speak to Us, and their feet will testify about what they used to earn.}   *(Yâ Seen 36:65)*

May Allah (swt) allow us to use our voices that day and may He permanently silence those who utter lies that lead to the silencing of our beloved ones.

One chance

Amr visited Rabaa Square two days before the massacre of August 14, 2013. Rabaa was full of men, women, and children holding a peaceful sit-in to protest the forceful removal of the first democratically-elected Egyptian president, Mohamed Morsi.

The morning after spending the night in Rabaa Square with some of his friends, Amr came home full of hope. He was impressed with the people he had met: their dedication to their cause, their generosity with one another, and their steadfastness in the face of what seemed to be insurmountable odds. He said to me, "I don't know what I'll do if anyone hurts them," as though he knew what was coming.

He was back in Alexandria when he heard that Egyptian security forces were advancing on the people in Rabaa Square and killing them. He paced back and forth in the apartment, tortured by his inability to help them. He cried in my arms. His gentle soul was so deeply grieved that he could not be consoled. I knew he wished he were with them but I was quietly thankful he wasn't.

Only two days later, he joined their ranks.

Not doing the right thing was never an option for Amr. He couldn't grieve over injustice and then simply move on the next day as we have been programmed to do. It was never an option for him to remain silent against oppression, to succumb to fear and hold back the truth in the face of intricately-woven lies.

I think he understood better than I that he only had one chance, one life, one soul.

You don't have infinite opportunities to do the right thing. The timer in your chest that is your heart is not just pumping blood through your body; with every beat it is counting down to the day you will return to the One to Whom you belong.

If we truly believed we have only one chance at rectifying our souls through worshiping the Creator, there would be urgency in all our thoughts, on our tongues, and in our limbs. We would be rushing, racing, doing all we could to get ahead. We wouldn't compromise the truth for fear of being harmed. We wouldn't be silent.

Doing the right thing would be our only option.

I grieve for myself, for the parting of a person most beloved to me. I do not grieve for Amr, though. He rose to the challenge and never stopped pushing forward in the race towards paradise until his final breath on this earth.

{Race toward forgiveness from your Lord and a garden whose width is like the width of the heavens and earth, prepared for those who believed in Allah and His messengers. That is the bounty of Allah which He gives to whom He wills, and Allah is the Possessor of great bounty.}
(al-Ḥadeed 57:21)

My Lord does not forget

On the night of August 15, one day after the brutal Rabaa massacre, I put Ruqaya to sleep in our Alexandria apartment and flipped open my laptop. I watched the horrific videos showing the bodies in Rabaa Square strewn everywhere, afflicted with unspeakable injuries.

I've never been able to watch those types of graphic videos – I don't have the strength or the stomach – yet I kept watching: insisting on knowing the truth, insisting on knowing exactly what happened and the extent of lives lost.

When I couldn't take it anymore, I put my laptop away and started sobbing into my pillow out of sheer disgust and pain. Amr woke up beside me and tried to comfort me. I kept telling him, "All those people in Rabaa were just like us. They look exactly like you and me." For the first time in my life, I wasn't watching bloodshed that was happening somewhere far from home. This was here. This was us.

I told him words that I will never forget: "I keep seeing your face on their dead bodies." I couldn't shake the despair. I couldn't shake the feeling that those countless rows of men whose bodies were lined up motionless in the morgues and mosques all looked to me like Amr.

He comforted me and told me not to worry. The next day was Friday, though, and the last time I saw him was as he was leaving for Friday prayers. Then, just like that, he was gone from my world, joining the ranks as a martyr, *in sha'Allah*.

It's strange to think that *years* have passed since then. Sometimes it feels as if it were just yesterday that Amr was standing in front of me with a smile so large and genuine that it made the hearts of those around him swell with happiness.

Even if a hundred years pass and everyone on earth forgets, my Lord is not forgetful. May the perpetrators of such crimes and all those supporting them see the punishment of Allah before their eyes and be unable to escape it.

May Allah (swt) have mercy on all those taken in those gruesome days and the many days that followed. May He enter them into His paradise where no eye will shed tears, no heart will be broken, and no fear will touch them.

May we be strong enough, unwavering enough, loyal enough, brave enough to also be honoured with the status of martyrdom.

Betrayed by a brother

In the weeks leading up to August 16, Amr attended a few peaceful anti-coup protests in Alexandria. He would walk with the protesters for awhile in solidarity and then come home. In those days I remember telling him, "Never raise your hand to hurt anyone. Don't even lift a rock from the ground and throw it at the 'security' forces. If you find people fighting each other, leave."

I advised him with these words because I was worried for the state of his soul. I didn't want him to mistakenly engage in anything that could cause Allah (swt) to be displeased with him.

In reality, I had no reason to worry. Amr never raised his hand against anyone. In one instance when he found some protesters clashing with security forces, he immediately left because he knew that wasn't the path to justice and reconciliation.

In light of this, I often reflect on these verses:

{And recite to them the story of Adam's two sons, in truth, when they both offered a sacrifice [to Allah], and it was accepted from one of them but was not accepted from the other. Said [the latter]: I will surely kill you. Said [the former]: Indeed, Allah only accepts from the righteous [who fear Him].

If you should raise your hand against me to kill me – I shall not raise my hand against you to kill you. Indeed, I fear Allah, Lord of the Worlds.

Indeed I want you to obtain [thereby] my sin and your sin so you will be among the companions of the fire. And that is the recompense of wrongdoers.

And his soul permitted to him the murder of his brother, so he killed him and became among the losers.}

(al-Mâ'idah 5:27-30)

Amr *never* raised his hand to hurt anyone, but his "brothers" in nationality raised their hands to kill him. In the end, those who have killed are the losers in the sight of Allah.

The light of Allah

Amr was shot through his chin and the bullet exited the back of his neck with a downward trajectory, meaning he was shot from a high place. He was likely killed by an army sniper.

They shot him through his beard – the one thing that differentiated his appearance from many others – as if to say: *Be humiliated for being the kind of Muslim we don't approve of; the kind who is true to the word of Allah, even if it's difficult; the kind of Muslim we find dangerous because he won't let injustice go without speaking up.*

The sniper picked him out of the crowd because of the ideals that he was assumed to represent. Even when his soul was already gone from this earth, they still couldn't leave him and his loved ones alone. At his burial in the graveyard, state-sponsored thugs viciously attacked the mourners with knives and rocks, hurling a rock that scraped me across my face. They wanted to humiliate us further.

What they don't realize is that we are not the humiliated ones. Rather, they are the ones who will be debased for their actions.

Try as they may to cover up their evil crimes; try as they may to silence people by murdering and imprisoning them; try as they may to quell the light of Allah – Allah (swt) will perfect His light and expose them on the day there is no Protector except Him.

{They want to extinguish the light of Allah with their mouths, but Allah will perfect His light, although the disbelievers dislike it.}   *(aṣ-Ṣaff 61:8)*

I cannot give in to fear. I continue to write because I cannot let them win by remaining silent. I know that those who are truthful will be separated from those who attempt to cover the truth.

Hold fast to your belief in Allah (swt) and know that He will always perfect His light.

Allah's invitation

Amr wasn't at home here in Canada.

He sorely missed the boisterous and close-knit Egyptian way of life. There was always a mosque at your doorstep, friends were close by, and neighbours actually knew one other. Here, he felt disconnected.

He was happy to visit Egypt again, to be close to the people and places he loved most. However, a few weeks into our visit things took an ugly turn. Strangers began harassing him in the street simply because he was bearded. They assumed, solely based on his appearance, that he was of a certain political stripe. People he respected and loved among his family and friends were supporting murder and oppression.

There he was in a place he thought was home, feeling like an outsider even amongst those he loved. He was a wanderer in those days, caught between two lands, neither of which invited him to feel at home. I could see this inner struggle bearing heavily on his heart.

So Allah (swt), the One Who is most merciful to His slaves, relieved him of this struggle and called him back to his true home. In doing so, He has invited me to remember the direction of the straight path that leads to my true home, too.

When the world becomes narrow, Allah (swt) invites you to seek the home that is expansive. When life becomes painful, He invites you to seek a life in the place that has no sorrow or grief. When you lose hope in people, Allah invites you to open the doors of hope in Him.

The rise and fall of oppressors

The man I love is under the ground and the regime that was the cause of his murder is thriving, its leader sitting on a presidential throne. It's strange that he thinks he's won. Doesn't he know that the higher an oppressor rises in worldly status, the greater his fall will be?

{And never think that Allah is unaware of what the wrongdoers do. He only delays them for a day when eyes will stare [in horror].}   *(Ibrâheem 14:42)*

Oh you who have stolen my love and removed happiness from the hearts of his parents: fear the day when you will have no weapon to defend yourself, no armour to protect you, and nowhere to hide.

Stepping stone

When the sadness of oppression weighs heavily on your heart as though a boulder were placed upon your chest, do not let it crush you. Push it aside, force it to bend to your will, and use it to as a stepping-stone to climb closer to your Lord.

As for those who have oppressed you, thank them. In the process of damning themselves, they have placed at your disposal a means for you to gain nearness to your Lord.

Counting tears

At one-and-a-half years old, Ruqaya was proud of herself. She would hold up a picture of our family, point to me, and say, "Mama!" Then she would point to herself and say, "Rakeeka!" (she couldn't say her name just yet). Then she would point to Amr and say, "Baba!"

Baba.

I don't count my tears. They are quickly wiped away; they evaporate from all surfaces and are merely a thing forgotten. Amr's parents don't count their tears. Ruqaya's tears are still part of the unknown.

But the Day of Gathering is coming. Allah (swt) will bring forward all creation, unite souls with their bodies once more, and make us stand before Him to be judged. That day, there is no moment in life that will not be revisited. We will see everything, our memories sharp with every transgression we have ever committed.

Every tear that was cried in public or private, under the cover of night or in the light of day, will be counted. I pray that our tears are gathered that day, every single one of them becoming a witness against the ones who unlawfully took Amr's beautiful life.

May the oppressors of the world drown in the tears of those whom they have wronged. May they taste the bitterness of what their own hands have earned.

{There is none in the heavens and the earth but comes unto the Most Beneficent (Allah) as a slave.
Verily, He knows each one of them, and has counted them a full counting.

And every one of them will come to Him alone on the Day of Resurrection (without any helper, or protector, or defender).} *(Maryam 19:93-95)*

May Allah (swt) grant us patience, which is better for us than what we have lost.

The death of humankind

{...whoever kills a soul unless for a soul or for corruption [done] in the land – it is as if he had slain mankind entirely. And whoever saves one – it is as if he had saved mankind entirely...}   *(al-Mâ'idah 5:32)*

When I stood by Amr's body, looking down at the man who had not let go of my hand from the moment we married until the day he left this world, I felt as though the "humankind" that I once knew was dead.

Allah (swt) describes it in this verse exactly as it feels: when they killed Amr, it felt like they had killed everyone. They killed every hope, every dream, every moment of happiness, and every genuine smile. They almost killed my faith in people doing the right thing.

Amr was just one man amongst billions of men, but to me he was everyone.

Holding onto hope

Evil has touched my life in a way that will always remain with me. I wish my daughter would never have to find out about this evil, but with time and maturity I know she will come to understand what happened to her father.

I do not look forward to seeing that look of pained understanding in her eyes.

When I feel overwhelmed by the evil I see in this world, I remember this verse:

{And [mention, O Muhammad], when your Lord said to the angels: Indeed, I will make upon the earth a successive authority. They said: Will You place upon it one who causes corruption therein and sheds blood, while we declare Your praise and sanctify You? Allah said: Indeed, I know that which you do not know.} *(al-Baqarah 2:30)*

Before our species was even created, the angels knew that evil and bloodshed would come from our hands. When they asked Allah (swt) why He would create humans, He simply answered:

{...I know that which you do not know.}

Allah knows that among us there will be men and women who are true to their promises to Him. Although there is great evil, there is also immense good in people. How can I not have hope in humanity when Allah (swt), Who knows everything, still has hope in us?

I pray to always be someone who fulfills her obligations to Allah (swt). I pray to always have hope.

True parenthood

A few months ago I heard a story of an Egyptian mother who had a son in the army. When she realized the army might go out and kill innocent protesters at Rabaa Square and other places in the summer of 2013, she called him and said, "I would rather see you imprisoned for life for failure to obey orders than know you have killed a single innocent person. I would rather cry over your dead body than know you have unlawfully taken a believer's life."

This is a serious statement. Those who refuse to obey the orders of their army leaders can easily be imprisoned, tortured, and even killed. She knew that was a possibility for her son if he failed to obey an order. As a mother, she understood how painful her life would become if she really did lose him.

I don't know anything about this woman. I don't know her name, her son's name, or where in Egypt she lives. I know only of her incredible statement to her son. I think about her often and I think about what her statement means to me as a mother.

What sets her apart is her unwillingness to sacrifice her son's position with his Lord in order to ensure his physical safety. Many parents want to keep their sons and daughters physically safe by any means necessary, regardless of the consequences. A parent who understands the true purpose of this existence, however, would rather see his or her child perish in this world for the sake of Allah than to know he or she is "safe" but has earned the anger of Allah.

{O you who believe! Ward off from yourselves and your families a fire (hell) whose fuel is men and stones, over which are [appointed] angels, stern [and] severe, who disobey not [from executing] the commands they receive from Allah, but do that which they are commanded.}

(at-Taḥreem 66:6)

May Allah guide us to be parents who always understand the higher purpose.

Blindness of disbelief

Pharaoh and his army drowned in the sea. He saw every sign and miracle that Allah (swt) gave Moosa (as), culminating with the greatest and clearest of them all: the parting of the Red Sea.

Upon reflection, it seems strange that he and his army drowned. I say "strange" because he saw with his own eyes that an entire sea had parted to make way for Moosa (as) and the Children of Israel to pass. Wouldn't that cause him to step back for a moment and think: *Perhaps there is a Lord who is aiding Moosa. Perhaps I am wrong. Perhaps I should be afraid of this unseen, ultimate Power*?

Such are those who are stubbornly arrogant, those who delight in the oppression of others, and those who continuously refuse to see the miracles and signs of Allah. Even if the greatest sign of all were to come to them, they would walk past it into oblivion as if blind.

O Allah, grant us the ability to *see*.

The ground will be opened

Most of those who are guilty of oppression and murder walk free. They nonchalantly pull triggers and snuff out lives deemed "unimportant." They use their power as politicians, police officers, and judges to imprison people who are innocent yet they allow those who have committed egregious crimes to walk free. They travel the earth like Qaroon, lost in their inflated perception of self-worth.[39]

They forget that the ground split open and swallowed Qaroon.

Every soul shall taste death and so, too, will the ground be opened for the oppressors as they enter their graves. When they are judged in front of Allah, they will have no speechwriters to help them twist the truth and eloquently present their cases. They will have no police force or military standing behind them, ready to come to their defense.

They will have nothing except their bodies: their weak, mortal, made-from-clay bodies, standing before *al-Hakam*, the Judge.

Their mouths will be sealed and their limbs will speak the truth. Those who were oppressed will finally receive true justice that will take into account every tear, every pang of sorrow, every moment of darkness that the oppressor caused. Nothing will be forgotten that day.

Nothing.

How we long for Your justice, our Lord! How, too, we fear Your justice if we transgress against ourselves.

Allah's Plans

{…But they plan, and Allah plans.
And Allah is the best of planners.}

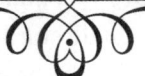

Allah's plans

August 17, 2013 was the date we had set for our daughter's *'aqeeqah*. We wanted to gather the people Amr and I loved in order to celebrate Ruqaya's arrival.

Indeed, the people we love did gather that day. They came in droves; they came in the hundreds. It was not to celebrate, though.

August 17, 2013 became the date of Amr's funeral.

We plan. We plan it all. We map out our happiness and success and make five-year goals, ten-year goals. We plan our careers before we graduate from high school. We plan our weddings before we get engaged. We choose our baby names before we get married. We talk about every country we want to visit and how we'd love to make a million bucks. We expect to live until we're a hundred.

Amr was twenty-six, tall, sturdy, smart, healthy. He was never touched by major illness or in any serious accidents. He was intelligent and hard-working. All indicators pointed to him living a long, productive life.

Except for one thing: when Allah (swt) created the pen and ordered it to write, it wrote that he would live for twenty-six years and one month. It wrote that he would be removed from this worldly existence in the matter of a few moments on August 16, 2013.

So it was. The angel of death is a dutiful servant. What we plan all falls away in the face of Allah's ultimate plan.

In the days and months after Amr left this world, I felt like death was near me. I smelled its coppery blood scent everywhere I went. I felt its grip, as though its fingers were being wrapped around my throat. I wrote my will. I felt like I would only exist here for a matter of days, then die like Amr.

Now I sometimes forget what it feels like for death to be so close to me. I forget and I make mistakes and say and do things that I later regret. When I am finally shaken out of that state of obliviousness, it hurts. It hurts to remember that I'm just a human who will err and fall and have the dirt of sin accumulate on me.

I can do nothing but hinge my hopes on Allah (swt) the Pardoner, the Merciful, the Forgiving, the Eternal Refuge. I hope that when the time comes for me to meet Him, He will forgive me not because I am perfect but because I tried to be a better version of myself every day and because I admitted my weaknesses in His presence but wasn't too arrogant to seek His help and forgiveness.

Today could be my last day. These could be my last words. The bullet of death isn't reserved for people of a certain age or geographical location. It will hit me. It will hit you.

At different stages in life, people often say to one another, "Don't worry. You still have time."

I say something different: *worry*. You have no time.

The Opener

When Allah (swt) decrees that a door in your life is to be opened, no matter how hard you try to close it, no matter how far you run away from it, it will remain open until you walk through it.

When Allah (swt) decrees that a door is to be closed, no matter how many times you knock on that door, try to break it down, or cry on your knees in front of it, begging it to open again, it will never be opened.

Grieve in front of the closed door if you must. Stand there for a time and look at it. Memorize its shapes, its lines, and its indentations. Hold your hands over your heart and press down to calm its quickened, pained rhythm.

Then know – know beyond the shadow of a doubt, know in your heart of hearts – that when you trust Allah and walk forward, He will open a more beautiful door for you. You will walk through it and perhaps you will even praise Him for having closed the past door you loved so much.

He is *al-Fattah*, the Opener. May the doors He opens for us always lead us back to Him.

Darkness and light

Staring into the sunset over the Mediterranean Sea was one of Amr's favourite things. I have many photos of him with his eyes lost in the rhythm of the waves. Sometimes we would watch the sunset together; sometimes he would go to the seashore alone. When the edge of the sun was close to the horizon, he would fall silent, watching the blazing orange sun as it dipped itself into the sea, slowly descending until the last ray disappeared from sight.

I didn't realize that while we watched the sun set together, the sun was also setting over our life with each other.

When Amr was killed, the sun set and the darkness of the night scared me. I was alone, walking blindly on the edge of a dangerous precipice over the sea. I could still *hear* life; I could hear the crashing waves, the rhythm of time moving forward, the laughter and chatter of people. But I couldn't *see* life.

At first I was scared of the darkness but soon my eyes adjusted to the lack of light. Soon I realized that beneath the stormy waves were expensive treasures and the only way to retrieve them was to dive straight into the nighttime sea. It would be difficult and it would require a kind of courage that I had never employed before.

I knew the treasures would be worth it.

If the sun never set on our happiness in this world, perhaps we would stand on the shore, motionless, dazzled by the sun's warmth and splendour. Maybe we would never have looked down into the darkness of the sea. Maybe we would not have dived into its depth to retrieve the treasures of patience, faith, and constancy.

Every sunset has its purpose. Every sunset reminds us that this life is waning, escaping, disappearing before our eyes. It reminds us that there are both light and darkness in this existence, both happiness and sadness. It reminds us that nothing is stationary.

Through the ups and downs, the darkness and light, the depth of pain and the elation of joy, the faith in our hearts can never set. When darkness surrounds us, the light of guidance within our hearts is what casts a thin stream of light, illuminating our path forward.

Prophet Muhammad (saws) said:

"How wonderful is the affair of the believer, for his affairs are all good, and this applies to no one but the believer. If something good happens to him, he is thankful for it and that is good for him. If something bad happens to him, he bears it with patience and that is good for him."[40]

Alhamdu lillah for the darkness.
Alhamdu lillah for the light.

Divine mercy

I love my daughter, almost to a fault. The crinkle of her eyes when she laughs, the way her lips curve downwards when she is asleep, the new words she learns daily, the mischief she always seems to get into: I love her; I love it all. She reminds me of her Baba, may Allah have mercy on him.

Sometimes I make decisions that cause her distress. I take things away from her that I know will cause her harm. Not everything is a toy, not everyone is a friend. It hurts me to see her tears, but she doesn't understand that my knowledge is greater than hers and I only wish to protect her. I only wish to raise her to be a better person than me.

Allah (swt) takes from us, too.

He takes the people we love the most. He allows people to usurp our wealth. He allows our safety to be shaken and our homes to be demolished. Yet He is still more merciful to His slaves than I am to my child. His knowledge is greater than ours. His planning is more perfect than ours could ever be.

What is the value of a home or wealth or safety when they cause us to forget Him? What is the purpose of having those we love close to us when it makes us complacent? If He wishes good for a people, then perhaps a painful disease that will actually bring about greater healing is better than lasting health.

When we see our world falling to pieces and our thought-out plans becoming nothing more than scattered dust, it's easy to succumb to that distressing question: *Why is Allah doing this to us?*

Don't succumb.

We would be wise to remember Allah is more merciful to us than a mother is to her child, in every circumstance, in every moment – even those moments when the pain is so sharp that it feels as though your heart will be split into two.

Especially in those moments.

He is ridding you of sins you may have forgotten about and is giving you the opportunity to raise your hands to the sky to seek His forgiveness. He is paving the road for you to walk the same path of great struggle that our righteous forefathers once walked.

He is strengthening you for your task.

A mother's love is the most powerful worldly love. It causes her to sacrifice her own soul so that her child can live another day. It makes her go hungry so that her child may eat. It makes her leave all her own hopes and dreams behind so that she may water the seeds of hopes and dreams in her child.

Still, Allah is more merciful than her.

Not knowing the future

How merciful our Lord is that He did not allow us to know the future. How many of us would shy away from our dreams if we knew we would fail? How many of us would escape the idea of love if we knew we would have our hearts broken? How many of us would not study, have children, or embark on a journey if we knew these things would bring us much pain?

We would live small, simple lives. We would never try, never climb, never soar.

Had I known Amr would no longer be with me less than three years into our marriage, had I known the intensity of the pain and the loss, had I known how empty the world would seem without his love – had I known, the fear in me would never have allowed me to marry him.

If I hadn't married him, though, I wouldn't have known how far this depth of love could go. I wouldn't have had Ruqaya, who astounds me every day with her sweetness, love, and endearing imperfection. I would have lived a safe life, but small and without light, without joy.

I've heard many people lamenting over their situations saying, "If only I had known," but if you had known what hardships would come, you wouldn't have ever striven to do something and be someone better. You wouldn't have done anything at all. You would have sat at home, feeble and crippled by fear.

Yes, the pain hurts. The failure stings. The impact of your fall has injured you deeply. You may look into the mirror and no longer recognize yourself from the wounds that now line your heart.

Healing is beautiful, though, and success comes after failure. When you are at the bottom, you learn how to build upwards better than before. You may not know it now, but the awkward and imperfect scabs and scars on your heart make it beautiful.

How merciful our Lord is that He does not let us know our future. He is merciful to let us fail, merciful to let us lose, merciful to let us feel pain.

It is only because of this mercy that we are able to try and strive and attempt love and happiness.

Alhamdu lillah.

Allah responds

In the weeks before Amr was killed, the atmosphere on the street in Egypt became particularly hostile towards bearded men like him. I used to notice the unfriendly stares directed at him when we would go out together. I had a nagging feeling of worry. I consistently asked Allah (swt) to protect him.

I do not believe in a deity that does not respond to supplication.

I believe in Allah (swt), Who has promised to respond to *du'a*. I believe in *al-Mujeeb*, Who has said:

{...Call upon Me; I will respond to you....} *(Ghâfir 40:60)*

I believe in the One Who is always near to me:

{And when My servants ask you [O Muhammad] concerning Me – indeed I am near. I respond to the invocation of the supplicant when he calls upon Me...} *(2:186)*

If Allah (swt) promises to answer the *du'a* of the supplicant who calls on Him, then I know He answered my *du'a*: not because I am special or free of sin, but because Allah (swt) never breaks His promise.

I asked Allah (swt) to protect Amr, so it must be that Amr was taken from me in order to be protected from some pain or some trial that I, in my limited knowledge, do not understand.

When you ask Allah (swt) for something and He gives you the opposite, He is not rejecting your *du'a*. Rather,

He is giving you what is better for you although you may not perceive it.

My Lord, my foresight is so narrow. Although I cannot perceive it, make Amr's departure better for me.

Word for word

Sometimes people think their *du'a* will never be answered. They think: *What I'm asking is too far-fetched. I'm too sinful. There are too many barriers.* Don't they know that Allah (swt) is *al-Mujeeb*? He is the One Who responds, regardless of how difficult your situation seems.

I prayed for Amr to come into my life. Sitting in my room alone, I would make this *du'a* consistently: "O Allah, bless me with a righteous spouse who will bring me happiness in this world and the next, who will bring me closer to You and be a means of me entering paradise."

That was my *du'a*, word for word.

Then Allah (swt) gave me Amr. He brought me happiness in this world and he encouraged me to be closer to Allah (swt), both in life and in death. If I am patient through the difficult trial of losing him, I do not doubt that the Most Merciful will reward my patience with paradise. That is His promise.

Allah (swt) gave me what I asked: perfectly, exactly, and without much effort at all on my part. It's not that I was without sin or that there were no barriers. It certainly seemed to be a far-fetched *du'a* at the time. I wasn't making these requests of a feeble and weak human being, however. I was asking the One Who is able to do anything and He responded.

I asked Allah for a righteous spouse and He gave Amr to me.

I asked Allah for happiness and He gave that to me.

I asked Allah for paradise and He gave me this test to see if I am worthy. I pray that I am.

Far be it from Him to not give you what you ask or better. Far be it from a believer to not trust that He will respond to those who call.

Perspective

Life is a matter of perspective.

The rich man is envied for his wealth but if his loved one drowns in one of his grand swimming pools or chokes on an expensive and rare cut of meat, what will the rich man's wealth mean to him then? No abundance of gold coins can fill that trench of pain. The wealth that once brought him joy will turn to ash in his hands.

The poor man is envied by very few. The roof of his tiny dwelling leaks, he has faded and tattered clothes, he sleeps on a worn and creaky bed, and he goes from one unstable job to another, seeking sustenance for his loved ones. However, his loved ones are huddled around him, their smiles warming him on cold nights. The difficulties have made him grateful.

Every person on this earth has one thing in common: we do not rejoice in hardship or pain or suffering. We want our hardships to end. We wish for our days to be full of only love and laughter and abundance.

Yet when we stand in front of Allah (swt) on the Final Day and see how many of our sins were expiated because of the pain we were exposed to, we'll wish those difficult moments had lasted our whole lives. When we see the untold rewards that are reserved for those who remained patient in every difficulty, we'll wish we suffered every moment of every day in this world.

{And no soul knows what has been hidden for them of comfort for eyes as reward for what they used to do.}

(as-Sajdah 32:17)

Mount Sinai

The only mountain I've ever climbed is Mount Sinai. Amr and I went on a trip to the Sinai region of Egypt after we were married. We left our hotel in the middle of the night and began the ascent at around three in the morning. We were meant to reach the summit in time to witness the sunrise. Mt. Sinai is surrounded by other mountain peaks as far as the eye can see and their shadows loomed around us, black and heavy against the sky.

I was in awe of the thousands of stars that pierced the darkness. Being born and raised in the city, I had never seen stars like that. The view was both awe-inspiring and frightening.

Regardless of how many stars there were above us, the path ahead of us was completely dark. We were armed only with weak flashlights, unable to see more than a few feet in front of us. I couldn't see the top of Mt. Sinai because it was so dark. As the dawn light began to emerge and I was able to see just how high the mountain was, I told Amr, "If I had known the mountain was this high, I wouldn't have attempted to climb it."

Because I didn't know how difficult it would be, I tried. I just put one foot in front of the other and after much difficulty I was sitting at the top, surveying Allah's creation.

The darkness scares us. The fact that we cannot see except what is immediately ahead of us scares us. The faint, looming shadows of what *might be* scares us.

If we had stood at the base of the mountain of life in bright, unadulterated daylight and saw the path that led to the peak – the pain, the exhaustion, the scrapes and bruises – would we have ever climbed?

Light is a gift, but darkness is also a gift. The unknown is a gift. It gives us the courage to try. It gives us the courage to say every so often: *Perhaps it will be just a few more days until I reach the summit, perhaps another hour, perhaps just a few more steps.*

So it is that we cannot see what Allah (swt) has planned for us or when we will reach the summit. We do not know ahead of time that it will hurt, that we will be injured in the process, or that we will lose our fellow climbers in the night.

We *cannot* know. If we did, we would never climb. If we never climbed, we would never reach the summit and see the sun rise over Allah's creation, standing above the clouds and uttering an honest *alhamdu lillah.*

Trusting in Allah (swt) means that your feet keep moving forward even when you cannot see what is ahead. It's knowing that He will care for you, grant you the gift of courage to keep going, and never leave you to yourself even for the blink of an eye.

That is the light we need in the darkness of the unknown.

The cure

Whenever my daughter is sick and I attempt to give her a dose of medicine, she cries and tries to escape my grip. I find myself wishing that instead of protesting and trying to knock the medicine out of my hands, she would understand that taking this medicine is for her own good.

How can I expect that level of understanding from a baby, though, when the same happens with adults? When Allah (swt) gives us cures and remedies for the diseases of our hearts, we scream and cry. We hate the cure and push it away.

Every calamity, every pain, every bit of suffering could be the means of our purification. It could be our passageway out of obliviousness to *reality*, yet we desperately wish that things were different. We reject pain and we turn our backs on patience.

I wish I could always remember that the more bitter the medicine, the more beautiful and complete the cure.

Were it not that Allah treats His slaves with the remedy of trials and calamities, they would transgress and overstep the mark. When Allah wills good for His slave, He gives him the medicine of calamities and trials according to his situation, so as to cure him from all fatal illnesses and diseases, until He purifies and cleanses him. And then (He) makes him qualified for the most honourable position in this world, which is that of being a true slave of Allah, and for the greatest reward in the hereafter, which is that of seeing Him and being close to Him. *(Ibn al-Qayyim)*

Just one child

Ruqaya was only nine months old when Amr passed away. In their attempts to comfort me, many people said, "It's a good thing you only have one child. Imagine how hard it would've been if you had a few!"

At the time I didn't know how to respond, so I just gave them the standard smile and nod. Truthfully, though, one of the great sources of my pain came from the fact that I had always wanted to have many children with my husband; I had imagined at least four.

Every human plan is superseded by Allah's plans, though.

I often think about the wife of 'Imran, the mother of Maryam (as). She pledged the baby that was in her womb to the service of Allah (swt). When she gave birth to a girl instead of a boy, she said in surprise:

{...My Lord, I have delivered a female. And Allah was most knowing of what she delivered...}   *(Âl-'Imrân 3:36)*

She had assumed that she would give birth to a boy who would grow into a strong man and have the ability to serve Allah. Instead, Maryam's mother gave birth to the best of all women, whose service to Allah caused her to be a revered role model long after her departure from this earth.

Then Maryam gave birth to the honoured messenger, 'Eesa (as). May Allah be pleased with them all.

Allah (swt) knew what the wife of 'Imran wanted. She wanted to serve Him through the service of her child. She dedicated the unborn child to Him. In accepting this act of worship from her, Allah (swt) gave her these *two* blessings in her lineage instead of *one*.

I love to reflect on this story because it illustrates the great generosity of Allah (swt) in that He takes our actions, our pledges, our devotions and He multiplies them according to whatever He wills. In turn, when we ask only of Him, He grants us what we ask or better.

We should all hold onto that great and beautiful hope in Allah. Even if we are able to have only one child or we have children that aren't exactly who we were expecting – or no children at all – we shouldn't dwell on it. Perhaps Allah (swt) will give us the blessings we seek (and better) in another form, at a later time.

I have hope in Allah's generosity. Instead of mourning the children that I never had, I've redirected that energy into continuous *du'a* for the child I do have.

I raise my hands and ask Allah (swt) to guide her and to bless her and her offspring in innumerable ways. Then I lay my hands back in my lap and silently hope that one day she will be better for me than ten children would have been.

I trust that from her, from this little three-year-old who drives me up the wall, much good will come to the world. After all, Prophet Muhammad (saws) told us the supplication of a parent for his/her child will never be rejected.[41]

We are given blessings in every possible form. We are even given blessings through pain. We ask Allah for happiness, stability, wealth, children, and health and He tests us by taking them away or delaying His response. Sometimes the pain that is left in the absence of what you desire is the soil that your heart needs to grow.

His ultimate plan is absolute in perfection.

He didn't give you exactly what you wanted because there is something better. Perhaps deprivation is better for your soul. Perhaps there is something more blessed coming. There is always a plan; of that there is no doubt. The only doubt lies in whether we will open our eyes to see it.

Brevity

{…You stayed not but a little –
if only you had known.}

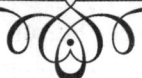

Graveyard

The silent, narrow pathways of graveyards help you to understand the brevity of life. There is little noise there – perhaps just the wind rustling through some lone trees and the faraway chatter of gravediggers who have taken a break from their work. Perhaps there are the muffled cries of the deceased's child or wife. Perhaps your own nervous heartbeat thuds loudly in your chest and ears.

The graves are full of people who were great conversationalists, talented writers, illustrious cooks, and fashion idols. They all met the same end.

What shade of lipstick matches your outfit doesn't seem to matter when you walk those lonely pathways. Your sharp mind that often wins word-wars with others doesn't seem to be able to bring itself to say a word as you touch the soil beneath your feet, the soil above their heads. The expensive shoes that are covered with the dust of that hushed graveyard don't seem so valuable anymore.

Everyone who existed before has died. Everyone who exists will die. The breath in your chest as it rises and falls is an indication that time is passing. Every moment gone is a piece of your one chance: *gone.*

At death you will not wonder: *What would my life have been like if I had more things?* You will not wish to have made more money or to have been more fashionable. You will not wish you had more degrees to your name.

You will only wish that you had worshiped Allah better. Only that. Nothing else.

The angel of death stands by, unbeknownst to you, as your time nears its end. He makes mourners of merry people. He obeys the orders of Allah without fail, without any choice in the matter.

One day it will be me under the soil. One day it will be my loved ones wiping their tears and walking with hushed words away from where I am. One day I will wish that I had worshiped Him better. I will wish only that. Nothing else.

That day it will be just my deeds and me. I fear that perhaps I will not have done enough. Perhaps the angel of death will take me before I am ready to meet my Lord, before I have given away my money to those who had a right to it, before I have decided to give up everything that leads me away from the path of truth.

Restlessness, then, is what I seek: tired eyes and worked hands. I seek until the day I am deposited into the graveyard to never rest until I have given everything I can, worshiped Allah with every limb of my body, and carried others through their difficulties.

Restlessness in this life is what I seek. The time for rest will come soon.

The living and the dead

Every autumn, I am reminded of the thin line between life and death. I am reminded, too, that among the animated bodies of those who are living are those who are already dead. Among the still bodies of those who are dead, there are those who are actually still alive.

Our hearts pump blood into our limbs. Our limbs are able to move and take us from place to place. Our eyes see. Our mouths speak. Our ears listen. By every physical marker, our bodies are alive. Some of our hearts are already dead, though.

It is strange how sometimes we mourn deeply over the loss of our beloved ones. We cry, we seclude ourselves from the world, we feel a sadness so dark that even the radiant sun cannot bring light to our hearts. How many of us mourn our beloved ones who are still physically alive but spiritually dead? That is the true death.

Ibn Taymiyah[42] said, "Remembrance (of Allah) is to the heart what water is to the fish. And what is the state of a fish that leaves the water?"

We are a people satisfied with granting sustenance to our bodies, adorning them with the best clothes, and scenting them with the most fragrant of perfumes. If we could only see into our sputtering and struggling hearts, we'd be met with the stench of rotting corpses. Our hearts are dying while our bodies are living.

Call it what you will, but this isn't *life*.

There are those who truly and meaningfully live: those who remember Allah standing, sitting, and on their sides;[43] those who have taken their share of this world, strengthened and sustained their bodies only so that their hearts may first live here and then move on to live the eternal life.

How beautiful the state of the believer whose heart has been truly alive in this world with the remembrance of Allah and who is blessed with eternal life under the protection, mercy, and forgiveness of Allah.

The inevitable

Those who have died now know the reality but can no longer do good deeds. Those who are alive can do good deeds, but they do not really *know* the reality.

Every soul shall taste death. I have not yet tasted it, but I have touched it. It's cold. It turns food and drink into ash when it enters your mouth. It nests in the pit of your stomach, churning and eating away at the edges of your being. It also removes doubt in the inevitable destination.

When the burden of life is heavy, so heavy that you feel your knees are about to buckle and the muscles in your hands have seized up from carrying this weight, you may look towards the ground and wonder if dying would be easier than this.

People wish for an end to pain, but they don't really wish for death. At least they wouldn't if they knew what would come after. Not if they knew that they would be alone – utterly and profoundly alone – beneath the soil, with only their belief in Allah and good deeds as protection. Not if they knew they would be able to hear the footsteps of those they love leaving them behind to fend for themselves.

Allah's Messenger (saws) said:

"Let none of you wish for death. If he is righteous then he might increase his good deeds, and if he is sinful then he might repent."[44]

Do not wish for it, but know that the inevitable will come and it will not stop to ask for your permission.

When your head goes down in prayer and your forehead touches the ground, know that this is the same ground in which you will be buried. Stay there, breathe in the scent of the earth, dig your hands into it, and make it familiar to all your senses. It will certainly become your home, for a time.

The last time

On December 23, 2010 Amr's friends ambushed him, picked him up, and threw him into the air several times outside the mosque to celebrate our wedding. On August 17, 2013 those same friends silently carried his shrouded body to where he would be placed in his grave.

We had just started our lives together and we were making the kinds of plans everyone makes for a family, a home, a career. Then suddenly, it was all over. When I spoke to Amr on the phone just a short while before he was shot and killed, it never crossed my mind that it would be the last time I would hear his voice, his laugh, or his "I love you."

You never know when "the last time" will be for you to do or say anything. The angel of death is a dutiful servant to his Lord; he will not pause or wait if it is your appointed time.

{Say: Indeed, the death from which you flee – indeed, it will meet you. Then you will be returned to the Knower of the unseen and the witnessed, and He will inform you about what you used to do.} *(al-Jumu'ah 62:8)*

Fix that which you have broken, join that which you have unlawfully separated, remember your grave often, remember Allah often. Make amends. Make amends. Make amends. Do not be fooled into leaving this world before Allah is pleased with you and before your loved ones hold you in high esteem and pray for you.

My Lord, witness that I hold Amr in high esteem! Grant him Your love, take charge of his family, and guide us to the path of truth, compassion, and sincerity that we may also be enveloped in Your mercy that knows no limits.

Who is this good soul?

The eyes roll up at the moment of death, following the soul as it is emptied from the body. It is the moment we fear, that which we loathe, what we would give all our riches to avoid: death.

I saw Amr in a similar state after he was killed. I remember his body and face resting motionless, the blood that had dried on his face and beard. It wasn't really him anymore – just the shell that had once housed his soul. I remember those tears as I stood over him wondering what my life would be like after losing a love so great.

The prospect of meeting death makes our hearts recoil in fear. We face death daily, seeing pictures and videos of victims of war shared widely on social media and in the news. Death came to them as a decree from their Lord. The pictures are gruesome; the reality even more so. We see devastated parents standing over their children's bodies and women standing over the remains of their beloved husbands. It's truly one of the hardest things anyone will have to face in this life.

Many faces of the dead have one thing in common: their eyes are still open. They are open because they have seen what we have yet to see and tasted that which has not forced itself upon our senses: death.

We ought to remember that as gruesome as it looks and as much as our stomachs turn in disgust and anger at the perpetrators of war crimes, the souls of our dead are now free. The men and women who truly believed in Allah and stood tall in the face of injustice have had their sins wiped clean at the first drop of their blood.

That which looks gruesome to us was perhaps a most beautiful experience for them.

Prophet Muhammad (saws) said:

"When the believer is about to depart from this world and go forward into the next world, angels with faces as bright as the sun descend from the heavens and sit around him in throngs stretching as far as the eye can see. Then the angel of death comes and sits at his head and says: Good soul, come out to forgiveness and pleasure from Allah! Then his soul emerges like a drop of water flows from a water-skin and the angel takes hold of it.

When he has grasped it, the other angels do not leave it in his hand even for the twinkling of an eye. They take it and place it in a perfumed shroud and a fragrance issues from it like the sweetest scent of musk found on the face on the earth.

Then they bear it upwards and whenever they take it past a company of angels, they ask:

Who is this good soul?

and the angels with the soul reply: So-and-so the son of so-and-so, using the best names by which people used to call him in this world. They bring him to the lowest heaven and ask for the gate to be opened for him.

It is opened for him and angels who are near Allah from each of the heavens accompany him to the subsequent heaven until he reaches to the heaven where Allah the Great is.

Allah, the Mighty and Majestic, says: Register the book of My slave in *'Illiyoon* and take him back to earth.

I created them from it and I return them to it and I will bring them forth from it again…"[45]

To have beautiful angels wrap you in sweet-smelling shrouds, call you by your most loved names, and take you into the company of Allah, the Most High: that is the definition of success.

I often wonder what Amr was called by the angels as they were lifting him to his meeting with Allah. I hope they called him Abu Ruqaya as he loved his *kunyah* greatly.

When we look at the countless gruesome photos coming out of war-torn countries, we cry because we think the people have suffered greatly – and they *have* suffered! But look where our beloved ones are now. Look at how they have been freed from the darkness and distress of this world into the light and pleasure of the hereafter.

We are the ones imprisoned. We are the ones who are still not safe. They, on the other hand, have won.

They are free.

Brevity

If you knew you only had a day or half a day to live, what would you do?

The People of the Cave slept for 309 years, yet they thought they only slept for a day or part of a day:[46]

{And similarly, We awakened them that they might question one another. Said a speaker from among them: How long have you remained [here]? They said: We have remained a day or part of a day...}   *(al-Kahf 18:19)*

Our lives are just a few pieces of time strung together, like the period of time between the rising and setting of the sun. We do not have an abundance of tomorrows to fulfil our debts or our promises.

If you ask anyone, "Do you feel like you have lived a long life?" the response will most likely be, "It all passed by in the blink of an eye," even if he or she has reached a hundred years of age.

On the Day of Judgment, Allah will ask:

{... How long did you remain on earth in number of years? They will say: We remained a day or part of a day; ask those who enumerate.}   *(al-Mu'minoon 23:112-113)*

The truth is, each one of us lives on a precipice that is becoming dangerously narrower with each passing moment. The angel of death approaches us; our appointed time to die will not miss us.

This world is just a minute, a moment, a speck of dust in the grand scheme of time and eternity. The time that has already passed will not be brought back for you to relive. Make that minute you have one of worship, one of righteousness, one of kindness, gentleness, and courage.

{...You stayed not but a little – if only you had known.}
(al-Mu'minoon 23:114)

Time passes

{By time,
Indeed, mankind is in loss.}   *(al-'Aṣr 103:1-2)*

One of the only constant things in this world is that time will pass, as it has always done. It will pass at the rate and speed it has always passed. A minute is sixty seconds. An hour is sixty minutes. A day is twenty-four hours.

Time cannot be physically held. It cannot be rewound, slowed, or stopped.

The passing of time to one person can mean seeing his or her child grow, blossom, and become beautiful. The passing of time can be the vehicle through which one gains wisdom and knowledge. It can see someone encounter the peak of a journey that has taken a lifetime to complete.

To some, the passage of time helps heal deep wounds. To others, time intensifies pain or causes disease and old age to ravage the body and heart. The passage of time can see a person fall from grace after years of righteousness and commitment. Time can unravel what was once whole.

Time seems to "fly" when you're having fun, but seems to inch forward slowly at times of embarrassment, pain, heartache, and boredom.

We never have enough time, but simultaneously we have so much of it that we seek out activities to "kill" time.

Some seek to rewind time and live in the past. They concoct anti-aging technologies and search for fountains of youth. They worship trends so they don't seem old and dowdy. However, they can never win against that which pushes forward, regardless of their sad, misdirected wishes.

Those who win are those who accept that they cannot stop time and use each hour to be better and do better than in the hour before.

How strange that time is and has always been consistent and yet used so differently by each person. A minute is sixty seconds. An hour is sixty minutes. A day is twenty-four hours. Within that time, some reach the pinnacle of existence through worship, generosity, and courage. Others dither away their valuable moments and have nothing except regret to reflect on.

Allah (swt) is the Creator of time and He is free from imperfection. He is the One Who caused it to begin and the One Who will cause it to end.

{By time,

Indeed, mankind is in loss,

Except for those who have believed and done righteous deeds and advised each other to truth and advised each other to patience.}   *(103:1-3)*

The reality of death

Death is treated with a forced sterility in some of the Western world. We hold our noses, wear masks, quickly whisk away bodies in specialized vehicles lest anyone be forced to see a corpse. We paint the faces of the deceased with makeup so we may remember them as they once were instead of as they currently are. Bodies are lowered into graves after the mourners have left to "protect" them from the shock; many people have never seen the inside of an actual grave.

We are removed from death, so we do not really understand it.

I remember when I entered the hospital morgue to see Amr a final time before he was buried. He was still in his clothes, his face still stained with some blood. One of the things I noticed immediately was that he was covered with a heavy blanket that looked familiar to me. It was a mixture of light and dark brown with a flower pattern on it. I thought it was strange because it was so similar to the one he used at his parents' home in the winter.

I recently happened upon a picture of a doctor who died in an Egyptian prison after being denied medical care. His body lay motionless on his bed, his grieved wife embracing him. I noticed that he was wrapped in a shroud that was just a thin, regular bed sheet bearing intricate flower patterns.

The things we happily purchase and use in our daily lives become the things we use on our dead. You may soon be wrapped in the bed sheet you sleep on. Your body and face may soon be covered with the same blanket you now huddle under for warmth.

Outside the Western parameters that espouse an unnatural obsession with separating life and death, the dead are often transported in regular family cars, being held close on the laps of those who love them.

The dead are carried on the shoulders of men, not just silently transported in thick wooden coffins. These men carry on their shoulders someone who was once alive, beautiful, and thriving. They see death, they touch it, then they put the body into the ground and watch as it is sealed in darkness upon darkness.

It's frightening, but it's the truth. It's only when you can really see it, touch it, and breathe its scent that you know it's coming for you, too. Every soul shall taste death.

It's a concept we hate to think about, an idea we do not want to approach until we reach old age. In reality, nothing about death is clean or palatable. We are not as far removed from it as some will have you believe.

We love our bodies but bodies perish. If only we loved our eternal souls and feared for their well-being as we fear for our bodies, we wouldn't fear death as we do. We would understand that it is messy and painful but necessary. It is necessary to die so we can truly live.

Our Lord, bestow upon our hearts concern for that which is lasting over that which will perish.

In the Shade
of Faith

*{…My Lord, build for me near
You a house in paradise…}*

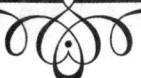

In the shade of faith

Faith is the only shade from the scorching heat of life's calamities. You will not find shelter outside of faith when the desert sun is at its peak, bearing down and pushing you into the dusty ground. You will not find a drink cooler than reliance on Allah when your throat is dry and your breathing is laboured. You will not find a resting place on this difficult journey safer than the piece of ground on which you pray.

You need belief in Allah more than your lungs need air. You need hope in His mercy and trust in His wisdom more than your heart needs to keep beating. You need His remembrance more than you need your limbs, your eyesight, or your hearing.

You need to worship Him more than you need to be alive. What is the purpose of life – the purpose of the air in your lungs and the blood pumping through your veins – if the essence of your soul is already dead?

The Prophet (saws) said:

"He who remembers his Lord and he who does not remember his Lord are like the living and the dead."[47]

Subhan Allah
Alhamdu lillah
La ilaha ill-Allah
Allahu akbar

We made it

Imagine entering the gates of paradise hand-in-hand with those you love. With your first step into your new life, angels greet you with beautiful greetings of peace. You have already forgotten every ounce of pain, sorrow, and frustration you have ever felt. It's nothing more than a distant dream now.

You are clothed in the softest silks and led by the angels through vast gardens of beautiful trees and plants growing succulent fruits. You are told that all these gardens and what is in them belong to *you*.

When you reach your home, you are amazed; it's bigger than any house you've ever imagined, more beautifully decorated than homes of the richest kings and queens. Its floors are made from hollowed pearls.

You recline on beautiful cushions, admiring all that Allah (swt) has given you and enjoying the musk-scented breeze of paradise gently caressing your face. You look at your companions whom you loved for His sake in this life and say to them: *We made it.*

{And those who are patient, seeking the countenance of their Lord, and establish prayer and spend from what We have provided for them secretly and publicly and prevent evil with good – those will have the good consequence of [this] home – Gardens of perpetual residence; they will enter them with whoever were righteous among their fathers, their spouses, and their descendants. And the angels will enter upon them from every gate, [saying]:
Peace be upon you for what you patiently endured. And excellent is the final home.}   *(ar-Ra'd 13:22-24)*

Towards His light

Al-Ahad filled the depravity in these bones with
    the sweetness of faith.
He replaced this hopeless heart
with a live, beating one
that believed divine relief was just a few steps in the distance.

In the night I cried out to Him,
Ya Allah, Ya Allah!
I ask you by all the names you have revealed in Your Book…

And He gave me the hardships He knew I could shoulder.
He gave me pain to expiate my sins
and so I loved Him more,
though my heart was heavy with grief,
and my shoulders slumped from the weight of sadness.

Now every gust of wind that blows against my skin
satiates my limbs with the desire to meet Him
and causes my eyes to close in sweet thought
about how a cool breeze in paradise would feel,
how it would evaporate the lines of age and distress
    from my face.

Ya Allah, Ya Allah!
My Lord, I am in anguish
that I replaced Your love in my heart with the love
    of people and things
believing they would make me whole
but they disappointed my heart and left it barren.

Ya Allah, Ya Allah!
I ask you through Your name by which if you are asked,
    You will not reject Your servant…

And He gave me more difficulties,
but I withstood them
and I stood taller, bending my face towards His light.

Now I wait for these moments, days, and years to pass
until I meet my Lord,
until I am able to bask in the brilliance of an everlasting rest,
until my heart is so full of love that it knows nothing else.

Ya Wadood!
Allow me to enter Your paradise.

No barrier between you and Allah

You aren't more difficult to see than a black ant, scampering over a black rock, under the cover of the darkest of moonless nights.

You aren't more difficult to hear than Yoonus (as) was when he cried out in the belly of a whale, in the blackness and depth of the sea.

What is inside you isn't harder to know than every single leaf that changes colour and falls off of every autumn tree.

Allah (swt) sees you, hears you, and knows what is hidden so deep within yourself that it may still be a mystery even to you.

He can distinguish your quiet whispering voice from the voices of billions of others. The bustling of marketplace shouts and arguments do not drown you out. The roaring of stormy oceans do not drown you out. Your voice doesn't crackle or get cut off when you're calling out to Him. This isn't a long distance phone call.

Your suffering isn't unknown to Him. Your anger isn't unknown to Him. That which you've suppressed and controlled within you isn't unknown to Him. The truth of everything, though you may be hiding it from everyone else, isn't unknown to Him.

There is never a moment when His seeing, hearing, or knowledge fail.

Why, then, do you seek to be seen or heard or understood solely by His creation whose seeing, hearing, and knowledge fail all the time? They can't see what's behind the external, can't hear except that which you say out loud, and can't understand that which you have protected with fortresses within you. No matter how much you desire for others to understand your secret self, there will always be a barrier between you and them.

Everyone is hiding something. If all that is hidden is known only to Him, it must follow that true contentment and true ease and true peace can be sought only at His door.

Submitting

Your body already obeys Allah, even if you don't worship Him.

Even if your forehead has never touched the ground, even if your tongue has never uttered a single phrase of remembrance, even if the mention of Allah causes you to cover your ears – your body and your world obey Him.

Every atom in every cell, every organ, every spurt of blood that is purified by your heart and sent back into your bloodstream are obeying His command. The moment He orders them to stop, to slow, to fail – they will.

Every moment you live through, every breath of air you take in, every thought that has ever crossed your mind was already recorded far before you made your entrance into this world.

There is nothing in the heavens and the earth that is not bound by His laws, by His ultimate decree. Not even you. Your heart and mind can never be forced to worship Allah, but they cannot escape obeying His commands.

If only we would obey His commandments consciously, too.

{The day the shin will be uncovered and they are invited to prostration but the disbelievers will not be able,
Their eyes humbled, humiliation will cover them. And they used to be invited to prostration while they were sound.}

(al-Qalam 68:42-43)

Strangers

Those who strive are strange, they are few, and they are far between.

The Messenger of Allah (saws) said:

"Islam began as something strange and will revert to being strange as it began, so give glad tidings to the strangers."[48]

The people in this world and that which they have engineered to distract and numb you from the reality are a strong current. You, the stranger, are swimming against this formidable tide. Sometimes you are strong enough, faithful enough, and confident enough to push forward. Sometimes, in moments of weakness, you are swept away.

When you are a stranger in a world full of close-knit friends, a traveler in a world full of those who are sedentary, relieve yourself for some moments from the burden of strangeness and the strain of journeying.

Take rest, weary soul, in reflecting upon that which will make you feel at home, among friends: the trees which bow with you in prostration at the command of their Lord, the birds chirping His praises, the mountains that would crumble into dust if the words of Allah were to be revealed to them,[49] every cell and nerve in your body: they all submit to their Creator.

Everything exists in the form He created and willed; everything does as He commands:

{Do you not see that to Allah prostrates whoever is in the heavens and whoever is on the earth and the sun, the moon,

the stars, the mountains, the trees, the moving creatures, and
many of the people?...}   *(al-Ḥajj 22:18)*

Perhaps you are strange amongst people with minds
that are constricted, that deny, that defy the existence of
Allah and vilify those who obey Him. You are not strange
amongst all other creation, though. While externally you
may feel that you are struggling, you exist in peace with all
creations in the heavens and on the earth.

Sit with the moon, sit underneath the shade of a silent
tree that has been alive longer than you. Listen to the wind,
to the melodious birds. Walk through the rain and retrieve
washed-away flowers to examine that which blossoms. This
is another world.

Take your rest with those who do as you do: who
worship silently, who submit, who are anticipating a
meeting with the Most High. Soon you will have to regain
your strength and return to being strange.

Hiding from the light

When the light of faith tries to enter our lives, sometimes it hurts – like the first moment you emerge from a dark room into the sunlight. You squint your eyes and shade your face from the sun's intensity. Yet after a moment or two, you can see that whatever the light has touched has been brightened and beautified.

There are people who don't want the sun in their lives. They prefer the darkness and squalor of disbelief and oppression. They draw the shades and hide behind locked doors to get away from guidance.

If the rays of light still enter in thin and gentle streams to remind them that there is something better, they angrily board up the windows, seal every crack, and cover their eyes.

They'll do anything to get away from the truth, anything to get away from the light.

However, the moment of death will uncover their eyes and they will see what their reality is, whether it is one of mercy or punishment. Those who cover their eyes now will have the veil they placed upon themselves removed:

{And every soul will come, with it a driver and a witness. [It will be said]: You were certainly in unmindfulness of this, and We have removed from you your cover, so your sight, this day, is sharp.}　　　　　*(Qâf 50:21-22)*

What good is our eyesight here if we can't really see? What good is the breath in our chests if we can't really breathe? What good can possibly come of sealing ourselves in darkness?

It's time to let the light in.

The tree that never dies

The axe thinks it has won when it cuts down the tree.

Little does it know that these are trees unlike others. These trees have roots running so deep that they continue to feed the soil even after being cut down; branches extending so high that their death means only that they will finally ascend towards that which they were reaching; they bear fruits during all seasons and produce seeds that are scattered in the wind, their destinations and effects beautifully unknown except to Allah.

The trees are believers.

{Have you not considered how Allah presents an example, [making] a good word like a good tree, whose root is firmly fixed and its branches [high] in the sky?
It produces its fruit all the time, by permission of its Lord. And Allah presents examples for the people that perhaps they will be reminded.}   *(Ibrâheem 14:24-25)*

Although my beautiful tree is gone from here, having ascended to that for which he was reaching, his roots remain. His seeds remain. His fruits remain. The landscape is not barren! While the seeds left behind grow again into new, strong, beautiful trees, the axe will rust and be thrown aside, useless.

You see, the axe can never win against a tree that never dies.

Mercy over wrath

My daughter is convinced there are peacocks in paradise.

I'll tell you how this conversation goes. First she asks for her dad and I tell her he's in paradise. Then she says she wants to go to paradise, too, so she can see him. I tell her we will go and see him one day, *in sha'Allah*.

Then our conversation continues and takes on strange and interesting turns, with her enlightening me on the specific things she would like in paradise, including big lions and the ability to tickle these *jannah*-peacocks – and they will be required by law to laugh (I'm paraphrasing).

I laugh, but then I wonder at what point this love and wonder in our lives turned sour. At what point did we become so engrossed in fearing Allah that we forgot the beauty of His mercy and His reward? Why don't we think about the proverbial peacocks in paradise?

Prophet Muhammad (saws) said:

"When Allah created the creatures, He wrote in the Book, which is with Him over His throne: Verily, My mercy surpasses My wrath."[50]

A wise person said that if you continuously teach your children to fear something, they will want to stay away from that thing. If we continuously lecture them about fearing Allah's punishment, why would they make nearness to Him a priority?

If Allah (swt) Himself says that His mercy supersedes His wrath, then the right way to teach is mercy first, wrath

227

second. It isn't just an equal balance between the two because Allah clearly says one is greater than the other.

{...and never give up hope of Allah's soothing mercy: truly no one despairs of Allah's soothing mercy, except those who have no faith.} *(Yoosuf 12:87)*

So I would like to talk about mercy more. I would like my daughter to hold onto her wonder and limitless imagination. As she grows, I will tell her about the fruits and drinks of paradise, the trees, the homes, the cushions and thrones, the gardens: all created to inspire her to seek and to hope.

If she sincerely hopes to get there, perhaps she will also love to follow the commandments of Allah, that she may finally enter paradise. *In sha'Allah.*

Maybe there, among the cushions, the thrones, and the gardens, there will be a peacock for her, too.

The price of paradise

The price to enter paradise is *you*. You give away everything you have, down to your life, to get in.

From deep within your soul, give love and hope and prayers for others. Every moment of time spent with your child, spouse, or loved one is you giving away that which is precious to someone you hold dear.

When someone needs your help, don't say "no" even if you're tired. When someone needs some of your wealth, don't say "no" even if you aren't rich.

Give from your skills and talents to make your community a better place. You are unique and someone somewhere needs you. Cook for your friends and send a container of cookies to your neighbour. Don't ask for the container back.

Put your life on the line fighting for good. Your life doesn't belong to you anyway; it belongs to Allah.

When you become so fatigued from giving everything away that the circles under your eyes have darkened and your shoulders have become hunched with the weight of the work, take a moment of rest to nourish your soul and strengthen your body. Then get up and give more.

The time for prolonged sleep and rest will come soon.

Don't hoard yourself and your things for too long because at the end, you will not be asked: *How much did you accumulate?* Rather, you will be asked: *How much did you give away?*

{Indeed, Allah has purchased from the believers their lives and their properties [in exchange] for that they will have paradise...}   *(at-Tawbah 9:111)*

The prick of a thorn

As humans, we are often unable to apply several different characteristics at one moment. For example, in moments of anger we may lose our ability to be merciful. When in love, we can be unjustly biased in favour of those whom we love.

Allah (swt) is the opposite. He is all of His beautiful names and attributes at once. He never ceases being merciful, even when He is angered. He never ceases being just, even if it is against those He loves.

While I have been given a painful trial, I understand that Allah (swt) gave it to me out of His mercy. It may seem strange to think of it this way, but I have many sins and I believe the pain and sadness that seem to follow me through my nights and days are cleansing me of those sins.

If I have to endure pain in this life so that Allah (swt) will spare me pain in the hereafter, isn't that pain actually a mercy from Him?

The Prophet (saws) said:

"No fatigue, nor disease, nor sorrow, nor sadness, nor hurt, nor distress befalls a Muslim, even if it were the prick he receives from a thorn, but that Allah expiates some of his sins for that."[51]

A home in paradise

Asiyah was the wife of the most powerful man alive, the Pharaoh of Egypt. She willingly gave up the wealth, honour, and status that came with that social position to believe in Allah and His messenger.

Pharaoh ordered her to be tortured to death for her beliefs and as she faced her final moments in life, she did not curse her tormentors or plead for mercy. She didn't question her faith or offer her assailants wealth to end the pain.

She rose above it all and set her sights on something much greater and more lasting. She looked to the sky and said:

{...My Lord, build for me near You a house in paradise...}
(Taḥreem 66:11)

Amr and I both loved wide spaces. Sometimes we would walk by large, beautiful houses and dream together that one day we'd have a home that was inviting, spacious, and uncluttered.

My hope for that home in this world has faded, but the hope for a better and lasting home near my Lord is still alive.

When the pain and the spaces in this world seem too cramped and too limiting, I close my eyes and imagine walking through a peaceful green grove of palm trees leading up to a quiet home. It sits in a place where the brightness and beauty has caused all pain to evaporate from existence. Then I repeat Asiyah's *du'a*:

{...My Lord, build for me near You a house in paradise...}

There is no better release of pain than to imagine myself one day in a place, if Allah (swt) accepts me into His mercy, where I will be near the One Who created me, Who sustains me, Who comforts me, Who has more mercy on me than a mother has on her child.

This is why I must consciously exchange that which is fleeting for that which is permanent.

{What is with you must vanish: what is with Allah will endure. And We will certainly bestow, on those who patiently persevere, their reward according to the best of their actions.}   *(an-Nahl 16:96)*

Our meeting place

In addition to being continuously abused, ridiculed, slandered, and plotted against, Prophet Muhammad (saws) had to endure watching those he loved being tortured and killed in front of his eyes.

He used to pass the family of Yasir, Sumayyah, and their son, 'Ammar (rahum), and see them being tortured in the desert heat of Makkah. All he could do was say to them:

"Patience, O family of Yasir! Your meeting place will be paradise."[52]

When everything around me seems to be pushing me to lose hope, when I know that I can't do anything to alleviate the suffering of people that I love and respect, I remember this story. It makes me hope with every fibre of my being that our meeting place after pain, heartbreak, and separation will be paradise.

Then perhaps Allah (swt) will honour us and allow us to meet our Prophet (saws) who, through his own intense pain and sacrifices, taught us how to lift ourselves up and persevere, even in the face of seemingly insurmountable odds.

May the peace and blessings of Allah be upon Muhammad.

Blessings of a hardship

Sufyan ath-Thawri[53] said, "In our view, a person does not have an understanding of the religion until he thinks of a hardship as a blessing, and comfort and luxury as being a hardship."

Sometimes people think it's difficult to turn to Allah (swt) in times of hardship. They think it takes stamina and strength to stay steadfast in His worship when the world has pushed them into the narrowest of corners and the darkest of places.

This isn't completely true.

When you come to a point during a trial when there is literally nothing you or anyone else can say or do to lift the immense pain from your heart, turning to Allah (swt) for relief is your only choice. To turn to anyone or anything else in this time can only be a form of madness.

The true difficulty lies in turning to Him during times of ease. In those smooth times when everything seems to be going just perfectly according to your plans, it becomes easy to lose sight of the One Who sustains you. It becomes easy to forget that the enjoyment of this world is temporary.

Times of ease require a type of patience that is difficult to master: patience in abstaining from evil and patience in performing that which is good. It requires a kind of consciousness and constancy that is challenging, even to the strongest among us:

{And when harm touches man, he invokes Us, lying down on his side, or sitting or standing. But when We have

235

removed his harm from him, he passes on his way as if he had never invoked Us for a harm that touched him!...}

(Yoonus 10:12)

How strange that a hardship may actually be a blessing while ease can be the true difficulty! May Allah (swt) make us from those who are constant in both ease and difficulty.

Too big for this box

You don't have enough time to be afraid.

There isn't time in your day for you to worry about what isn't in your hands. You should be too busy flourishing in productivity to be preoccupied with thoughts that cripple your courage. There is no space in your heart for fear.

It is only Allah (swt) Who can protect us in this life and in the next. Fear of Him empowers you to be courageous enough to not fear His creation. Fear of all others will only debilitate you, cast you into the darkness of cowardice, and keep your hands, mouth and limbs from doing good and saying the truth.

Consider how Allah (swt) protected His prophets and slaves, even when they were put into situations where their physical safety was seemingly much at risk:

Allah kept Moosa (as) safe as he crossed the Red Sea, on foot, with an entire nation of people following him. Pharaoh drowned in the same sea, on the same path.

He kept Nooh (as) and the believers safe in the flood that drowned the disbelievers.

He kept Maryam (as) safe even though she delivered a baby alone under a tree, without another human soul to help her.

He kept Yoonus (as) safe beneath the darkness of the night, the ocean, and the belly of the whale.

He kept Muhammad (saws) safe although the people attempted to assassinate him, threw stones and garbage at him, boycotted him, slandered him, and attempted to hurt him in every way possible.

We can seek help from people and ask them to protect us. We can go to places that are "safe havens" or hide ourselves away from that which scares us. None of that will prevent the decree of Allah from coming to our doorstep. None of it will prevent our souls from departing our bodies at their appointed time.

If you die in a state of disbelief, if you are resurrected without being granted a spot under the shade of Allah's throne, if your mouth is sealed and your limbs witness against you, if you receive your book in your left hand, who can you seek help from then?

What good will your fear of people do for you then?

We spend our lives fearing what others will do to us if we speak the truth or insist on staying faithful to our beliefs and values. We are preoccupied with attempting to fit our bodies and souls into the suffocating boxes they have cut out for us. We know we don't fit into those boxes.

The truth is too big to fit into a box. Our hearts are too busy and full to stay confined. Our souls are owned by the King, not by His slaves.

You have only a few moments on this planet. You don't have time to be afraid.

Dreams that never end

Discovering a new dream after you have lost someone or something beloved to you is painful. The darkness of dreamlessness sometimes feels safer than attempting to find a new dream. The blackness nestles itself into your being and it becomes almost comfortable to put all your dreams on hold. It becomes comfortable to be *stuck* because the darkness reminds you that you once had something beautiful and full of light.

Darkness cannot be our home, though. Our hearts weren't made to live without the light of hope, of faith, of dreams. Like trees, our hearts need light to grow and survive. They need to grow roots so they do not fall in the midst of storms. They need to be watered by constant remembrance and faith.

The darkness, although sometimes comfortable, cannot be a home for us.

I was reminded recently that there is no "end" to beautiful dreams. All the *du'as* we make for a dream to come to fruition, for happiness and comfort and stability – none of these *du'a*s are ever really gone.

In His ultimate wisdom, Allah (swt) decrees the losses in our lives. He decrees that we must lose something in this world: wealth, lives, safety. It's the nature of this existence.

When we lose our dreams – the same ones we prayed for all those days, months, and years; the same ones we fought to accomplish; and the same ones we stayed up during nights to beg Him for – those dreams are never actually lost.

Prophet Muhammad (saws) explained to us that *du'as* are answered by Allah (swt) in one of three ways:

1. Allah (swt) gives us what we ask for;
2. He wards off something harmful that would have otherwise afflicted us;[54]
3. The "unanswered" *du'as* are granted to us in full and in a better form in the hereafter.

Surely, the third is the best answer to any *du'a*.

Even if a dream has gone, your prayers for that dream are never lost. Far be it from Allah, the All-Knowing, to forget what you have asked, even if you yourself forget as time passes. Perhaps Allah (swt) is saving those precious, fervently-uttered supplications for you in paradise.

How merciful a Lord to not forget and to grant us hope in the darkness of lost dreams!

Healing

*"The reward of every deed is known
except for the reward of patience,
which will be like flowing water."*

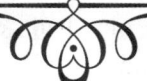

The sun still rose

The sun rose the morning after Amr was killed.

There was the darkness of pain within me: a darkness I didn't understand, a darkness that was all-consuming, and a darkness that sometimes still attempts to hold me hostage.

Still, the sun rose. I was almost surprised that it did. I couldn't understand how the day could be sunny and bright but simultaneously my heart could be bruised black and blue. I didn't want the sun in my life anymore. I wanted to close my eyes and not have to face light when everything inside me was pitch black.

The sun rose every day, telling me that time wouldn't stop to mourn with me. The world wouldn't stop to check if I was all right. The moon would go through its phases, the sun would rise and set, the weather would become cold, colder, warm, warmer. And repeat.

Nothing around me had changed even though everything within me had.

People sometimes ask me, "How did you move from day to day after what happened?" The truth is, I didn't move from day to day. The days used to move me. I was bound by the physical night and day. I was bound by my need to eat and sleep and wake and repeat. I answered those physical needs to survive because it was my only choice.

Time has allowed me to understand that it's a blessing that we don't have to make the days move forward. If the power to withhold ourselves from the light were in our hands, we would be stuck in the darkness of pain until we died. However, Allah causes the sun to rise to show us that we, too, will be moved forward.

The sun lays itself against our skin and tugs at us to rise from sleep. The light of guidance, too, beckons us to leave the shadows of pain and torment. It calls us to believe in a compassionate, merciful Creator. It calls us to deposit the pain within our hearts into the possession of the Lord Who heals.

{Say: Have you considered: if Allah should make for you the night continuous until the Day of Resurrection, what deity other than Allah could bring you light? Then will you not hear?}   *(al-Qaṣaṣ 28:71)*

Grief does not negate faith

In the days after Amr was killed, many people came to visit us at his parents' home in Alexandria. For almost a week, his parents' living room turned into a busy, messy space of muffled condolences and awkward tears. I knew a few of the visitors but most of them were strangers to me. The women hugged me, offered their sympathies and tears, then left.

One woman who came to offer her condolences looked at me with a wide smile and said, "There is no need to cry. Amr is a *shaheed*." I don't know who she was but I appreciated her conviction and the kindness in her eyes. At the same time, I couldn't help but feel that she was telling me to restrict something in myself that I couldn't possibly restrict.

Prophet Ya'qoob (as) lost his most beloved son, Yoosuf (as), when Yoosuf was just a young boy. Ya'qoob's pain never disappeared or waned, even many years after Yoosuf had disappeared. The grief was overwhelming, but he prescribed upon himself *sabrun jameel* (beautiful patience).

When his sons reproached him for his continuous remembrance of and sadness over Yoosuf's disappearance, Ya'qoob

{...turned away from them and said: Oh, my sorrow over Yoosuf, and his eyes became white from grief, for he was [of that] a suppressor.
They said: By Allah, you will not cease remembering Yoosuf until you become fatally ill or become of those who perish. He said, I only complain of my suffering and my grief to Allah, and I know from Allah that which you do not know.}   *(Yoosuf 12:84-86)*

Beautiful patience isn't a state that requires a lack of sadness; Ya'qoob went blind from the depth of his continuous grief, yet Allah never chastises him in the Qur'an for feeling this profound pain. He simply shows us how Ya'qoob dealt with his sadness: by complaining of his suffering only to Allah (swt) and seeking relief from Him. Even though he was a prophet and therefore knew with much more certainty that Allah (swt) would grant him recompense for what he had lost, his human emotions did not disappear.

On this path I am walking, I have sometimes felt absolutely broken to the point where I believed I could never hope in beauty, kindness, and happiness again. Then I pick up the Qur'an and read the story of Yoosuf (as) and his father, and the broken pieces of my heart slowly come together again, but not because the sadness leaves my heart. Rather, because I understand that sadness is a natural and undeniable part of the way the Most Merciful has created us. It's also natural for us to believe with every fibre of our beings that Allah will grant us relief.

Ya'qoob said to his sons:

{...despair not of relief from Allah. Indeed, no one despairs of relief from Allah except the disbelieving people.}

(Yoosuf 12:87)

Relief came for Ya'qoob. I know relief will always come for me, too, because the promise of Allah to His slaves is true.

Splint

Amr was my husband, my confidant, and my merciful and loving partner in life. After suddenly losing him, the loneliness I felt almost consumed me.

I was breathing a different kind of oxygen than everyone else. I was speaking a different language than my friends and family. I had turned a different colour, rusting and fading away. No one understood me and I understood no one. I may as well have been the only person on this earth.

Pain is alienating.

People often turn to the skies in search of some sign, some comfort, some explosion of reason to help them understand the tragedies of life, saying: *Please help me understand. Help me relieve this pain.* When their requests are not immediately answered, they return to the quietude of themselves, disappointed and broken.

As a response to this, I've often heard people say, "If you wonder where Allah is when you're going through pain, know that the teacher is always silent during the test."

This statement has no merit. The truth is that Allah has never been silent. He is not like the teacher who refuses to speak while the students are writing a stressful test. His words of guidance and healing are recorded in a Book that we can read any time we wish.

It is not He Who is silent. It is we who refuse to listen.

If we listened, we would know that Allah (swt) describes Himself as *al-Jabbar*; the Restorer, the Superb Comforter, the Healer of all wounds.

A word with the same Arabic root of *"jabbar"* is *"jabeerah,"* which is a splint that is used to set broken bones. Allah understands that sometimes we feel as though we are quite literally broken into pieces, troubled by the rattling sounds of those loose parts within us as we walk forward in this existence. He is the only One Who can restore what was once broken within us, transforming us so that our hearts are whole and sound again.

{O mankind, there has to come to you instruction from your Lord and healing for what is in the breasts and guidance and mercy for the believers.}   *(Yoonus 10:57)*

What is in your control?

Do not attempt to control your heart.

Your heart will be thrown down a well of sadness so deep that climbing out will feel impossible. It will be trapped under layers of darkness so black that light will seem like only a distant memory. It will become diseased and abandoned by all those who loved it. It will feel a pain so severe that it may wish to stop beating altogether.

Do not attempt to control your heart. You will fail.

Control your words instead. Say only that which pleases Allah; keep your tongue silent in the moments you feel you will say evil.

Control your body. Let your body do only that which pleases Allah; worship Him with your limbs and keep them from harming yourself or others.

Control your mind. Expose yourself only to good; abandon things that simply numb your senses or plunge you deeper into despair. Read, write, paint, work.

Your heart will eventually become that which you do with your body, your words, and your mind.

Don't assume that your heart is in your control. It isn't. Your body is, though. You choose what you will do, what you will say, who you will be. When you make the right choices accordingly, Allah (swt) will relieve your pain and guide your heart to a state of contentment.

Just as Yoosuf (as) was lifted out of the well, just as Yoonus (as) was saved from the belly of the whale, just as Ayyoob (as) was cured of disease and blessed with a loving family, and just as Maryam (as) was relieved of her pain and honoured – so, too, shall your heart be lifted, enlightened, cured, and relieved.

Patience

Patience comes only with great struggle and difficulty. You may succeed in holding onto it for a moment or two, but if you are not vigilant it will escape from your grip just as quickly as it came.

Patience doesn't mean to just "wait out" the pain. It doesn't mean burying your head in the sand until the storm has ended so you can safely re-emerge into life.

Patience isn't necessarily peaceful, at least not at first.

Patience is sometimes like stepping onto shards of glass and muffling your screams. As you sit and remove the pieces from your skin, tears stinging at your eyes from the pain, you smile and do not say a word.

Patience can feel like you're being lit on fire from within. You feel as if the fire will consume you. Yet you keep walking forward calmly, extending your hand to take cool drinks from those who offer them in order to quell the flame.

Patience is like treading water in violent seas after your boat has capsized. You are exhausted, but if you stop trying for a moment you will drown.

Part of Allah's mercy is that some of the believers who have been tried greatly in this world and who have remained patient will meet Him without any sins in their records at all.[55]

Patience does not mean that you do not feel or that you are unaffected by pain or loss. It isn't so now and it has never been. It's to wake up in the morning despite the pain and do what needs to be done to take care of yourself and your family.

You pray, you are punctual to work, you cook meals for your family, you smile and engage in harmless small talk about the weather, and you don't say except that which pleases Allah:

Alhamdu lillah: Praise and thanks belong to Allah

Inna lillahi wa inna ilayhi raji'oon: To Allah we belong and to Him we shall return

La hawla wa la quwwatah illa billah: There is no power or might except in Allah

Hasbuna Allah wa ni'm al-Wakeel: Allah is Sufficient for us and He is the best Disposer of our affairs

Tawakkalna 'ala Allah: We have placed our trust in Allah

Patience will extinguish the fire, lift the weighty burden, and lead you to dry land. This is not because you have been exceptionally good or are intrinsically worthy of being healed; rather, it is because Allah (swt) has promised:

{For indeed, with hardship [will be] ease.
Indeed, with hardship [will be] ease.}   *(ash-Sharḥ 94:5-6)*

I know that Allah (swt) never breaks His promise.

Allah's generosity towards the forgetful

Sulayman ibn Qasim[56] said, "The reward of every deed is known except for the reward of patience, which will be like flowing water."

Allah promises that He is with those who are patient[57] and they will receive a full reward without reckoning.[58] About those who remain patient at the strike of a disaster, acknowledging that they belong to Allah and to Him they will return, Allah promises:

{Those are the ones upon whom are blessings from their Lord and mercy. And it is those who are the [rightly] guided.}   *(al-Baqarah 2:157)*

Patience: its reward is heavy, blessed, and without limit because it's difficult. It requires vigilance, as though you are walking on a path filled with thorns. It requires that you live your life with a consciousness that you will return to the Owner of your soul. It requires you to not become distracted by that which is fleeting in favour of that which is everlasting.

We all become distracted, though. We all get cut by the thorns of impatience and sin when we have fixated our eyes on some momentary, frivolous thing. That is the nature of human beings; in fact, a word with the same root of the Arabic word *"insan"* ("human") is *"nisyan"* ("forgetfulness").

There is indeed pain in forgetting patience. There is pain in losing sight of our ultimate goal, even for just a short time. We cannot escape that which is our nature.

Prophet Muhammad (saws) said:

"I swear by Him in whose hand is my soul, if you were a people who did not commit sins, Allah would take you away and replace you with a people who would sin and then seek Allah's forgiveness so He could forgive them."[59]

Strange is the affair of the believer.

She is commanded to be patient and so she is and Allah loves her and is with her. Then she forgets because Allah (swt) has created her as a forgetful creature. Then she returns to Him in repentance for her mistakes, thereby affirming that He is the Lord who forgives; once again she attains His Love. As if that mercy isn't enough, He changes her misdeeds into good deeds.[60]

How generous a Lord and how sad is the state of the person who does not enter into Allah's mercy, which envelops all things.

A cure for loneliness

Loneliness cannot be cured by the company of people. A smile that has been disfigured by pain cannot be made well again by banal laughter. Eyes that have been pushed into the darkness of loss cannot see light again just because the sun is out.

The Keeper of secret pains, the Listener to hushed words, and the Knower of that which plagues the heart but is never spoken is your company when all other company loses its sweetness.

When the people have turned away from you and their presence brings you no comfort, choose to be in the company of the angels who witness.

The Prophet (saws) said:

"Verily the one who recites the Qur'an beautifully, smoothly, and precisely will be in the company of the noble and obedient angels..."[61]

When loneliness eats away at you and the company of others does not soothe the pain, seek the Highest Companionship.

Prophet Muhammad (saws) relates to us that Allah (swt) says:

"I am as My servant thinks of Me. I am with him when he remembers Me. If he mentions Me within himself, I mention him within Myself. If he mentions Me in an assembly, I mention him in a better assembly..."[62]

Recite the words of Allah (swt) and you are in the company of noble angels. Remember Allah (swt) in words and actions and He will be with you.

Do not look for the antidote elsewhere; you will not find it. There is no other cure for loneliness. There is no other relief.

{Those who believe, and whose hearts find rest in the remembrance of Allah. Verily, in the remembrance of Allah do hearts find rest.}   *(ar-Ra'd 13:28)*

Witness

I often ask myself in moments of grief: *Isn't it enough that Allah (swt) is a Witness over all things?*

When Moosa (as) was afraid that Pharaoh would kill him or reject him and his brother, Haroon (as), Allah (swt) said to him:

{...Fear not. Indeed, I am with you both; I hear and I see.}
(Ṭâ Hâ 20:46)

In another chapter, when Moosa explains that he is afraid Pharaoh will kill him, Allah (swt) responds:

{No. Go both of you with Our signs; indeed, We are with you, listening.} *(ash-Shu'arâ' 26:15)*

The beauty of this is that Allah's sight and hearing are not like our sight and hearing. We see and hear then forget or are unable to act upon what we have witnessed.

That which Allah (swt) sees and hears is not forgotten. He sees all – that which is apparent and that which is hidden – and will come to the aid of those who are fighting to hold onto patience and perseverance. He knows without having to be told or reminded and He raises the status of those who strive. He hears and responds to those who call upon Him again and again. That is a promise and Allah does not break His promises.

How comforting that it is Allah (swt) Who is with us, not just as a passive observer but as a Witness who will grant us support, peace, and tranquility in difficulty (with hardship, there is ease). He will bring forth all of our suffering for He has not forgotten, although others have. We will watch our evil deeds erased on the Day of Reckoning for the calamities that we bore with patience.

How can you abandon hope while knowing that when there are three of you, Allah is the fourth; when there are two of you, Allah is the third?[63] Even when you are by yourself, so alone that your heart feels as though everyone else has vanished from the earth, you aren't actually just one because He is there with you.

Moosa (as) was afraid! He was one of the greatest men to ever walk the earth, yet he was afraid. You, too, are human. Allah knows that you, too, are afraid. Moosa (as) was not chastised for his fear; rather, Allah (swt) responded simply that He was with him as a Witness, seeing and hearing. That statement was enough. It was enough to make Moosa and Haroon move forward on their journey with confidence.

I often tell myself: *It has to be enough that Allah is a Witness over all things, that He is the Keeper of secret pains and the Knower of the seeds of sorrow that are planted within the heart.* It is enough that He is with us, hearing and seeing the difficulties in our paths. It must be enough solace and healing to know that He is a Witness over all things.

{…There is nothing like unto Him, and He is the Hearing, the Seeing.}   *(ash-Shoorâ 42:11)*

No fear, no grief

Fear of an uncertain future and grief over a painful past are two ever-present emotional conditions that plague the human psyche.

Sadness over the past and fear of what the future may bring are two natural states that don't necessarily contradict faith. They are built into us but should be kept in check through knowing that Allah (swt) does not burden a soul more than it can bear and trusting that Allah (swt) has a precise and perfect plan for us.

Even then, the emotions still exist. This world causes us to continuously journey towards stations of happiness, but even when we arrive at these stations there are always memories of sadness or fears of future troubles quietly burning within us. Our lives in this world will never be free from fear or sadness.

The thing is, when you arrive at the final and greatest station of happiness – paradise – fear and grief will no longer exist.

Allah (swt) describes paradise as a place where believers will not fear nor grieve. From the start of human existence, these "emotional" rewards of paradise have been present. When Adam and Hawa' were expelled from paradise, Allah (swt) said:

{…Go down from it, all of you. And when guidance comes to you from Me, whoever follows My guidance – there will be no fear concerning them, nor will they grieve.}

(al-Baqarah 2:38)

When we think about the rewards of paradise, our minds automatically go to the tangible, physical rewards that can be seen, tasted, and touched: gardens, fruits, rivers of honey and milk and wine, beautifully-adorned homes, clothes of silk, and more. These rewards are beautiful and enticing and they fill our senses with anticipation. We shouldn't forget the other side of the coin, though: the reward of never having to feel fear or grief again; the reward of satisfaction, peace, eternal bliss, and reunification with the righteous of your family, friends, and the prophets and martyrs. This is the reward that is felt, not just seen or tasted or touched.

Allah (swt) mentions the reward for the believers of "no grief and no fear" over fifty times in the Qur'an. This is a sign of the utter perfection of Allah's design. While His rewards in paradise are beyond our comprehension, He tells us that they coincide with our every possible need and desire. Many of us desire, more than anything else, to not have to grieve anymore, to not have to fear anymore.

Allah (swt) knows that which plagues your heart of sadness and that which makes you fearful of the future. He is telling you again and again to strive for His sake, to believe in Him alone, and to follow the path He has outlined for you. He will, in turn, enter you into paradise, which is as vast as all the heavens and the earth.

There, no fear shall be on you ever again nor shall you grieve.

Darkness under darkness

Prophet Yoonus cried out to Allah from beneath three darknesses: the darkness of the belly of the whale, the darkness of the ocean, and the darkness of the night, saying:

{...There is no deity except You; exalted are You. Indeed, I have been of the wrongdoers.}   *(al-Anbiyâ' 21:87)*

No matter how deep the darkness in my chest is, how lost I am among the people, and how alone I feel, if I reach out in *du'a* to Allah He will hear me, He will see me, and He will help me.

Healing

My hope and trust are in Allah alone.

As He allows my skin to naturally heal itself with clotting blood, He will also allow my heart to heal. It is no matter that there will always be a faint scar there. The scar teaches me to never forget how He has healed me.

As He brings the night and day into being, as He causes the sun and moon to continuously exchange places each day, He will also cause my life to run its course exactly as it was meant to. I will never lose anything I was meant to hold. I will never hold anything I was meant to lose.

As He causes the earth to die, to be starved, to be deprived of any meaningful life, and then brings it back to lushness and beauty simply by saying "Be" – so, too, will He cause my body to die and disintegrate in the soil then raise me up and cause me never to die again.

When I placed my hope in people, they betrayed that hope. They took from me something that wasn't theirs to take. They injured that which was once healthy in me.

When I place my hope in Allah, I know that He will never betray His promise. He will return to me what I have lost, or better. He will heal my heart that has been struck open by the people.

So I say: I am satisfied with Allah as my Lord, Islam as my faith, and Muhammad (saws) as the final prophet. Only when this verbal statement of satisfaction truly enters the heart will it be able to heal. It is only absolute hope and trust in Allah, the Eternal Refuge, which causes the pain to subside.

Keep working

When Maryam (as) was in the throes of labour, her pain drove her to say:

{…Oh, I wish I had died before this and was in oblivion, forgotten.} *(Maryam 19:23)*

Allah (swt) shows us a response in the Qur'an that illustrates just a miniscule portion of His compassion and mercy. He does not chastise her but instead it is said to her:

{…Do not grieve; your Lord has provided beneath you a stream.} *(Maryam 19:24)*

What comes next is also key:

{And shake toward you the trunk of the palm tree; it will drop upon you ripe, fresh dates.
So eat and drink and be contented…} *(Maryam 19:25-26)*

She was instructed to shake the trunk of the palm tree. A woman who was giving birth and was experiencing so much pain and apprehension that she wished for death was now being asked to get up and shake a palm tree!

Those who have seen the thick trunks of palm trees know that to shake one is no easy task. Those who have gone through a painful labour and delivery know that simply standing up during or after it is difficult, let alone doing anything physically demanding. Maryam didn't collapse in pain or give up hope in recovery, though; she shook the tree and ate the dates that fell from it.

More than anything, this story has taught me that being in a state of pain doesn't exempt me from working hard. Now I stand up every day and I push all sorrow to the back of my mind. I write, I help with charitable causes, and I involve myself in projects that I believe in. Knowing that I'm able to work for the benefit of others and myself helps me understand that I still have a purpose to fulfil on this earth.

Allah (swt) promises relief, but He also orders us to do the work that needs to be done. Even if the pain of life has pushed you to your knees, you can never stop moving forward and working towards the next step on the path towards paradise.

Offering support

My daughter and I were once looking into a fish tank in a doctor's waiting room. She loves fish so we were both staring at them intently. I noticed a small fish struggling to swim. It would swim for just a few seconds and then get exhausted and start floating to the top of the tank. The poor creature looked as though it would die soon.

Then a larger fish positioned itself above the struggling fish and pushed it down so it wouldn't float to the top. Every time the little fish was nudged in this way, it would regain some energy and try to swim again. This happened over and over until we were called into the doctor's office.

When someone you know is about to float to the top of the tank – physically, spiritually, or emotionally – you need to nudge them back into health, faith, and hope. When someone needs you in a time of darkness and pain, hold them, relieve them, work with them until they reach better days. Even if they push you away and tell you they don't need your help, stay right there and make them swim.

Prophet Muhammad (saws) said:

"Whoever removes a worldly grief from a believer, Allah will remove from him one of the griefs of the Day of Resurrection. And whoever alleviates the need of a needy person, Allah will alleviate his needs in this world and the hereafter. Whoever shields [or hides the misdeeds of] a Muslim, Allah will shield him in this world and the hereafter. And Allah will aid His slave so long as he aids his brother…"[64]

I will never stop being grateful to the friends and family who visited me, brought me food, gave me their shoulders to cry on, and nudged me back into action when all I wanted to do was give up. May Allah remove from them all grief and worry on the Final Day.

Walk with me

My dear Ruqaya,

Walk Home with me, my cherub.

Stand next to me in the spot where Baba used to be and do not worry – I will carry you when you become fatigued and Allah will carry me when the burden is too heavy.

Hold onto me and don't let your grasp loosen. If you become lost in the chaos, come sit on my shoulders and look above the crowd.

Build with me a bridge to pass the pain and to patch our wounded hearts. Place the bricks with me, one by one.

Plant with me, my love, our gardens in paradise: *subhan Allah, alhamdu lillah, la ilaha ill-Allah, Allahu akbar*.[65]

There: I have given you the seeds. Hold them tight in your tiny hands until you're old enough to send them into paradise's soil.

Walk forward with me, my sunshine. We have only today to do the work that needs to be done.

The journey will end so soon and, *in sha'Allah*, tomorrow we will be Home.

Don't sleep through the pain

Two weeks before Amr was taken from us, I started a blog for Ruqaya so I could write letters and advice for her. Amr wanted to write on the blog, too, but he never got the chance.

This was my first message to her on August 3, 2013:

Dear Ruqaya,

My first baby, I carried you inside me for nine months and I thought you were a boy the whole time. We even picked out the name Bilal. The moment you were born and the doctor said, "It's a girl," I thought to myself: *But all the clothes I bought are blue!*

Well, you were my surprise and you still surprise me every day. I want you to have this place to come to in case I leave you one day. You might need something to look back on and remember who your mom was. Strive to be like me in the ways that I'm good and learn from my many mistakes.

Don't sleep through the things you need to experience to learn how to be a better and more patient person, even if it's easier to shut your eyes and ignore the pain. Be awake to the good things waiting for you in life, *in sha'Allah*.

This is for you, baby.

Love, Mom

Just two weeks after this, Amr was gone. As I re-read this right now, it seems as though the advice I wrote to her about not sleeping through the pain was actually advice to myself.

There is a kind of pain you should never sleep through. You should know it and it should know you. You should breathe it and let it sit in your lungs as though it will settle and breed and never leave. You shouldn't numb the pain with things that intoxicate the soul or try to fix it with clumsy school glue when you know it needs welding. You should let it almost crush you so that you may understand what rock bottom is.

If you never understand what rock bottom is, you'll never understand how great, how powerful, how merciful the One Who lifts you up from that bottom is.

Let Allah (swt) lift the pain from your heart. Let your eyes really *see* the beauty of a sunrise again. Let your heart really *feel* the unadulterated joy of your child's laughter. Let your ears really *hear* the chirping of crickets and birds as they praise Allah.

You see, if you keep fighting the pain and never let it in, you can never really let it out either.

Time passes

Allah (swt) is the Mender of broken hearts.

Time has passed since I got that most-hated phone call, since I stood over Amr's body at the morgue and tried to memorize every feature of his face before I would have to let him go, since we were attacked in the graveyard by people who hated the truth and righteousness that Amr stood for.

People wonder how I was able to hold myself together. They wonder why I haven't collapsed or given up hope in Allah or in the goodness of people.

I don't have an explanation from myself, but the answer can be found in the story of Prophet Moosa's mother in the Qur'an. She was instructed to place him in the water if she feared for his life at the hands of Pharaoh's army:

{And We inspired to the mother of Moosa: Suckle him; but when you fear for him, cast him into the river and do not fear and do not grieve. Indeed, We will return him to you and will make him [one] of the messengers.}   *(al-Qaṣaṣ 28:7)*

I often wonder about what kind of strength she must have possessed when she placed her infant child in a basket and pushed him into the water without knowing where he would end up. She did one of the most difficult things a mother could do. She held herself together with the help and guidance of her Lord and watched him drift away.

Moosa was accepted into the house of Asiyah, but he refused to breastfeed from any wet nurses. It was then that his sister, who had followed him, led Asiyah to take Moosa back to his mother.

What was the purpose of Allah (swt) returning Moosa to his mother? Moosa could have breastfed from any woman without returning to his mother. If it were so, he could still have grown up to be the messenger of Allah, his righteousness intact, his journey and story still remarkable.

There was a reason, though, that Moosa had to come home to his mother:

{So We restored him to his mother that she might be content and not grieve and that she would know that the promise of Allah is true. But most of the people do not know.}

(al-Qaṣaṣ 28:13)

Allah returned Moosa to his mother simply so that she wouldn't grieve, so that her heart would be at ease, and so that her faith would not waver.

Allah (swt) cared about this woman. He mended her heart, not so that the course of history could change or some big momentous event could take place. He mended it because He is merciful and loving to the believers. He mended it so that when we read her story we can know the extent of His love and mercy. That is all. And that is reason enough.

Allah (swt) doesn't wish for the believers to grieve and He wants them to know that His promise is true. I've lived it these past few years. Every time I was about to reach a breaking point in my despair or to fall into the darkness of losing hope, I would receive some news that would lift my heart. Someone would have a beautiful dream about Amr, someone would perform *'umrah* or establish some charity on his behalf. I would receive words of support from people I love and respect or encounter some verses in the Qur'an that would take me by the hand and hold me steady.

One day after I had finished the *'asr* prayer, about eight months into my widowhood, tears were streaming down my cheeks, my heart was aching, and I didn't know how to rid myself of this immense pain. I raised my hands to ask Allah (swt) to help me be able to somehow visit His sacred House to come closer to Him and for that to be a part of my healing. Before I was able to even make the *du'a*, my phone rang. It was Amr's parents calling me to tell me they were just at the Ka'bah making *du'a* for me to be able to visit it. I thought: *How strange that this prayer has yet to come from my lips and Allah (swt) has put the same prayer on the lips of people beloved to me in such a blessed place.*

My heart was lifted so much in that moment that the tears of sadness turned into tears of joy.

None of these things are coincidences. None of these things happened because I am particularly good or worthy. They happen because Allah (swt) cares about the hearts of His slaves. I know that He cares about me and about my daughter because I've lived in the realm of this immense mercy these past two years. Every ounce of pain was met with some inexplicable beauty and serenity that no human effort could produce. It was from Him. All of it.

If you believe in Allah alone with no partners or intermediaries and you worship Him alone and you sacrifice that which you love in order to come closer to Him alone, you will see wonders in your life. Your difficulties will become blessings. Your heartaches will become healing. Your *du'as* will be answered in ways that you could never have imagined. He doesn't want you to grieve and He wants you to know that His promise to the believers is true.

It's not any more complicated than that. It happened to me and it's still happening.

Alhamdu lillah.

Epilogue

About a year after Amr passed away, I was getting ready to move to another home when I made a curious discovery. Tucked away between some old clothes of ours, I found some strands of hair from his beard.

They stopped me in my tracks as I held them in my open palm. I trembled as I stared at the wildly long and curly strands. They were as black as they ever were.

Suddenly it was as though that one year apart from him had not passed at all. It was as though not even a day had passed. It made me think of all the days he would get ready for work, thoroughly brushing his hair and beard in front of the mirror, long strands of his beard falling to the ground and collecting dust, unbeknownst to him.

It was as if he had been in the room just before I had entered, brushing his hair to prepare for the day's journey.

The beard hairs weighed nothing. They were certainly worth nothing. Yet I knew at that moment that these few strands of hair were just about my most valuable possession. The first thing I did was go into the kitchen and put the hairs in a Ziploc bag. I pressed the air out of the bag and folded it several times. I zipped the bag into a pocket in my wallet that also holds our wallet-sized wedding photos.

In this moment of finding these stray hairs whose owner had long since been buried, I was reminded of the day of Amr's funeral. They reminded me that a year had passed since I had stood over him in the hospital morgue, looking at his face and stroking his thick beard in our final moments together. They reminded me of the snorkeling trip we took to the Red Sea and of Amr climbing back on board the boat, laughing, his beard dripping salty water.

They reminded me of walking, then running in the dusty graveyard where he was buried. They reminded me of the story of Moosa (as) and the parting of the Red Sea…

Allah (swt) ordered Moosa to escape from Pharaoh's grip with the Children of Israel under the darkness of night. They were pursued by Pharaoh and his mighty army who quickly caught up to them.

Moosa and his followers were standing with the Red Sea in front of them and Pharaoh's immense army behind them. His people panicked and said:

{…Indeed, we are to be overtaken!}

Moosa's response to them was:

{…No! Indeed, with me is my Lord; He will guide me.}
(ash-Shu'arâ' 26:61-62)

It was at this point that Allah (swt) inspired Moosa to strike the sea with his staff and made the sea split in order to make a way out for the Children of Israel.

When Moosa was put into a situation where he had to fully rely on Allah to make for him a way out, he told the people in full confidence:

{…with me is my Lord; He will guide me.}

Allah (swt) did guide him and make a way out for him.

At Amr's funeral, I waited until he was buried then made my way into the cemetery to visit his grave. Before I could get to his grave, we were attacked by state-sponsored thugs who heard there was a "Muslim Brotherhood" funeral going on (although this wasn't true). They ran after us, hurling stones and yielding knives.

I didn't see the faces of any of the men running after us. I didn't ever turn around. I knew they were there, though, because of the screaming of the women running directly behind me. I knew because I was hit across my cheek with a rock as I was running.

I was trapped. Behind me were these vicious men who had no reservations against attacking women. In front of me was a graveyard with extremely narrow and sometimes non-existent pathways. There was an older woman in front of me also trying to escape but having much difficulty running and climbing over tombstones to escape. There was nowhere for me to go. I was trapped.

When I think back to that moment, I nearly repeated what the Children of Israel said when they were trapped: *This is it for me. I'm going to be overtaken at any moment.* I had to remind myself that Allah was with me, seeing and listening. As I was struggling to climb over tombstones, I whispered a simple *du'a*: *My Lord, I know You are with me. Save me from this situation not for myself, but for the sake of my daughter who has already lost one parent.*

And He did save me. All of a sudden it was silent behind me, the pathway in front of me became wider, and Amr's friends who were ahead saw me and directed me to a quick way out of the cemetery.

I only later found out that the two women running right behind me whose screams were abruptly silenced were actually captured by these thugs. Although they were eventually released physically unharmed, they witnessed terrible things. If these men had caught me instead and found out I was the wife of the man they apparently hated so much, I still don't know what they would have done to me.

In those moments I knew I had no one to rely on except Allah, so He gave me a way out of that situation and many other situations since then. He sent me the people and circumstances to take my hand and lead me away from danger.

Allah (swt) promises:

{...And whoever fears Allah – He will make for him a way out. And will provide for him from where he does not expect. And whoever relies upon Allah – then He is sufficient for him...}　　　　　　　　　　　　　*(aṭ-Ṭalâq 65:2-3)*

Allah (swt) made a way out for me at that moment for a reason. The full reason is only known to Him and I am discovering small pieces of it on this journey.

Losing Amr meant I had to leave behind all my plans and re-evaluate my purpose in this world. His departure caused my life to swerve onto an unknown path. Many people have stumbled upon my writings in the past few years, captivated by the love Amr and I shared. These readers have walked with me on this new path, taking glimpses into the beauty of this love and the difficulty of this loss. They witnessed how, in the midst of the darkness, I had to learn how to unearth new dreams.

As Allah (swt) promises all believers, with this difficulty I have also experienced much ease. My daughter brings me joy every day. My family and friends have stood with me, holding me upright as I walked through this storm. My mind is full of ideas for exciting projects and initiatives. The sun still rises every day, casting its light and warmth on my daughter and me. The full moon still graces the sky and its unpretentious glow fills even the darkest of nights with whispers of hope.

Allah (swt) is the Most Merciful.

The few strands of Amr's beard hair that I had found tucked beneath some old clothes a year after his death were a significant discovery for me. Regardless of the ease Allah (swt) blesses me with I will still carry them with me wherever I go, not only because I love and miss my husband but because they remind me that someone who was so real and present was removed from this earth so quickly.

They remind me of the final moments I stroked my husband's beard before he was put into the ground. They remind me of the day of his funeral when Allah (swt) gave me a way out of a great difficulty.

They remind me that Allah (swt) gave me and continues to give me joy.

They remind me that every day I wake up with my soul still inhabiting my body and all my faculties intact is an opportunity to make decisions that will earn Allah's pleasure. They remind me that every day and every blessing is a gift from the Giver of gifts.

They remind me that nothing is permanent. Not even pain.

Acknowledgements

To my parents and family who have tirelessly taken care of Ruqaya and me with no questions asked: I thank you. My Lord, forgive me and my parents. Have mercy upon them as they brought me up when I was young.[66]

I thank my group of friends in Team Inspiration who comforted me in difficult times and encouraged me along this path of healing and self-expression. A special "thank you" is due to Hajera Khaja, who inspired me with the idea for this book in the first place.

Thank you to my editors, Shoilee Khan and Amina Sadler, who spent hours working alongside me to bring this book to fruition.

Thank you to my generous supporters, Nazia Nusrat Khan, Tariq Rafique, Ambreen Syed, Ieman Hassan, Shady Atta, Shahenda S., and Aaida Mamuji, for helping me make this book a reality.

Thank you to everyone who has ever secretly made *du'a* for me or sent me messages of encouragement and hope.

Notes

Bibliography

Ali, Abdullah Yusuf. *The Meaning of the Holy Qur'an*. New Delhi: Kitab Bhavan, 2001.

al-Hilali, Dr. Muhammad Taqi-ud-Deen and Dr. Muhammad Muhsin Khan. *Interpretation of the Meanings of the Noble Qur'ân in the English Language*. Riyadh: Darussalam, 1998.

Ibn Abi ad-Dunya. *As-Sabr wath-Thawab* 'Alayhi. Beirut: Dar Ibn Hazm, 1997.

Pickthall, Muhammed Marmaduke. *The Meaning of the Glorious Qur'an*. Flushing, NY: Tahrike Tarsile Qur'an, 2001.

Saheeh International. *The Qur'ân: Arabic Text with Corresponding English Meanings*. Jeddah: Dar Abul-Qasim, 1997.

Shakir, Omar and Arthur R. and Barbara D. Finberg, "All According to Plan: The Rab'a Massacre and Mass Killings of Protesters in Egypt." Human Rights Watch website. August 12, 2014. "https://www.hrw.org/report/2014/08/12/all-according-plan/raba-massacre-and-mass-killings-protesters-egypt" Accessed September 10, 2015.

Appendix:
Regarding 'Iddah

{And those of you who die and leave wives behind them, they (the wives) shall wait (as regards their marriage) for four months and ten days, then when they have fulfilled their term, there is no sin on you if they (the wives) dispose of themselves in a just and honourable manner (i.e., they can marry). And Allah is well-acquainted with what you do.} *(al-Baqarah 2:234)*

The limits a widow follows during the period of *'iddah* concern her vulnerable psychological state at a time when she has lost her closest support and may be in a state of shock. *'Iddah* pays respect to the late husband as well as protects the woman from exploitation when she may not be in a state to make major decisions or defend herself.

In some Muslim societies, *'iddah* becomes a prison. The new widow is told she is not allowed to leave her house at all, even for a breath of fresh air or to see a doctor. She is not allowed speak to anyone (even on the telephone), have a bath more than once a week, or brush her hair. Many such limits are not based on what is prescribed in the authentic sunnah.

According to authentic hadith, during her *'iddah* a widow is not to adorn herself with bright or decorated clothing (she is not restricted to wearing black or grey, however), jewelry, perfume, or makeup. She should not apply henna or dye her hair.

She is allowed do whatever she needs to do in her house: clean and take care of housework, cook food for herself and her guests, bathe whenever she wants, and speak to friends and family.

She should remain in her marital home but she may go out for legitimate necessities. She should be in the home before sunset, however, and should not spend the night away from the home she shared with her husband unless that home is unsafe. A recently-widowed woman also cannot accept a marriage proposal until the *'iddah* is finished.

Glossary of Arabic and Islamic Terms

adhan: the call to prayer that is recited prior to each of the five daily prayers

alhamdu lillah: all praise and thanks is due to Allah

Allahu akbar: Allah is Most Great

ameen: amen; O Allah, respond to what we have asked

'aqeeqah: the celebratory event held after the birth of a baby involving the slaughter of sheep and distribution of its meat to family, friends, and the needy

ash-hadu an la illaha ill-Allah, wa ash-hadu anna Muhammadun rasool-ullah: "I bear witness that there is no being worthy of worship except Allah, and that Muhammad is the Messenger of Allah;" the testimony of a Muslim's faith

'asr: the third prayer of the five daily prayers, performed in the late afternoon.

ayah: a sign; a miracle; a Qur'anic verse

baklava: a dessert made of thin pastry, nuts, and honey; common in the Middle East and Central Asia *du'a:* supplication

Eid ul-Fitr: the celebration marking the end of Ramadan, the month of fasting

fajr: the first prayer of the day, performed before sunrise

galabiyah/jalabiyah: an ankle-length garment often worn in North Africa and the Arabian Peninsula (it is also known as a *thawb* or *dishdashah*)

hadith: a saying or action of Prophet Muhammad (saws) that was narrated and recorded by his Companions and later generations

hajj: the pilgrimage to Makkah that all Muslims are obligated to make once in their lifetime (if they are financially and physically able)

hasbuna Allah wa ni'm al-Wakeel: "Allah is Sufficient for us and He is the best Disposer of our affairs"

hijab: clothing prescribed for Muslim women; in this text it refers to the head scarf

husn adh-dhann billah: having a good opinion of Allah or thinking well of Allah

'Illiyoon: a register in heaven in which good deeds of the pious are recorded

inna lillahi wa inna ilayhi raji'oon: "to Allah we belong and to Him we will return"

in sha'Allah: Allah-willing

'isha: the fifth and final prayer of the day, performed at night

istikharah: a prayer asking Allah to help one make a good choice

jannah: heaven, paradise

jihad: a struggle, either a war or struggle facing an enemy or a spiritual struggle within oneself

Ka'bah: the black, cube-shaped building at the centre of the Sacred Mosque in Makkah, Saudi Arabia; it is visited by millions of pilgrims each year. Muslims around the world face the Ka'bah while performing their daily prayers.

al-Kawthar: Prophet Muhammad (saws) said:
"[Al-Kawthar] is a river that my Lord has promised to me in which there is much goodness. And it is a cistern to which my nation will come on the Day of Resurrection." (Muslim)

kunyah: an Arabic epithet or nickname usually given to a person to signify and refer to the name of his/her first son or daughter (e.g., Abu Ruqaya means "the father of Ruqaya")

la hawla wa la quwwatah illa billah: "there is no power or might except in Allah"

la illaha illa-Allah: there is no being worthy of worship except Allah

mabrook: an expression of congratulations

miswak: a small branch used as a natural toothbrush

nikah: the official wedding ceremony

Qur'an: the Islamic sacred book, believed to be the word of Allah as revealed to Muhammad (saws) through Angel Jibreel

Ramadan: the ninth month of the Islamic calendar year in which Muslims fast from dawn until sunset

sabrun jameel: beautiful patience

shaheed: martyr

subhan Allah: "Allah is free from imperfection"

subhan Allahul-'Adheem wa bihamdihi: "glory and praise be to Allah, the Almighty" *sunnah:* the authentically-transmitted record of the teachings of Prophet Muhammad (saws)

tahajjud: night prayers performed after the time of the 'isha prayer and before the time of *fajr*

taqwa: being mindful of Allah; God-consciousness

taraweeh: night prayers performed in the month of Ramadan after the *'isha* prayer

tawakkalna 'ala *Allah:* "we have placed our trust in Allah"

'umrah: a lesser (non-mandatory) pilgrimage to Makkah that can be performed at any time during the year

wudoo: the ritual washing or ablution performed before prayer or touching the Qur'an

Grades of hadith appearing in this text

saheeh: sound; the most authentic level of hadith

hasan: reliable; one of the strongest classifications of hadith

hasan ghareeb: a reliable hadith which was narrated via only one chain and one narration

hasan saheeh: a reliable sound hadith

Names of Allah appearing in this text

al-Ahad: the Only One

al-Fattah: the Opener

al-Hafidh: the Protector

al-Hakam: the Judge

al-Jabbar: the Compeller; the Restorer; the Healer of all wounds; the Superb Comforter

al-Kareem: the Most Generous

al-Mujeeb: the One Who responds

as-Saboor: the Patient

ash-Shakoor: the Appreciative

as-Samad: the Eternal Refuge

al-Wadood: the Most Loving

al-Wahhab: the Bestower; the Giver

Endnotes

1   Shakir, Omar and Arthur R. and Barbara D. Finberg, "All According to Plan: The Rab'a Massacre and Mass Killings of Protesters in Egypt." Human Rights Watch website. August 12, 2014. "https://www.hrw.org/report/2014/08/12/all-according-plan/raba-massacre-and-mass-killings-protesters-egypt" Accessed September 10, 2015.

2   Amr was not from the Muslim Brotherhood; he was simply a religious man who believed in right and wrong, regardless of one's political leanings.

3   "I bear witness that there is no being worthy of worship except Allah, and I bear witness that Muhammad is the Messenger of Allah." This is the testimony of a Muslim's faith.

It was narrated that Mu'adh ibn Jabal (ra) said: I heard the Messenger of Allah (saws) say:

"If a person's last words are *la ilaha ill-Allah*, paradise will be guaranteed for him." (Ahmad; graded *saheeh* by al-Albani)

4   The Messenger of Allah (saws) said:

"Their (the martyrs') souls are in the bodies of green birds which have their nests in lamps hanging from the throne and they roam freely wherever they want in paradise, then they return to those lamps.

Their Lord looked down upon them and said: Do you desire anything?

They said: What could we desire when we can roam freely wherever we want in paradise?

He (Allah) did that with them three times and when they saw that they would not be left without being asked, they said: O Lord, we want You to restore our souls to our bodies so that we may be killed in Your cause again.

When He saw that they had no need, they were left alone." (Muslim)

5   Ahmad; graded *saheeh* by an-Nawawi.

6   at-Tirmidhi, who graded it *hasan*.

7   Muslim.

8   Ibn al-Qayyim al-Jawziyah (1292–1350 CE) was a celebrated Islamic jurist, commentator on the Qur'an, and theologian.

9   Narrated Anas ibn Malik (ra):

"We went with Allah's Messenger (saws) to the blacksmith, Abu Sayf, and he was the husband of the wet-nurse of Ibraheem (the son of the Prophet [saws]). Allah's Messenger (saws) took Ibraheem and kissed him and smelled him and later we entered Abu Sayf's house and at that time Ibraheem was in his last breaths, and the eyes of Allah's Messenger (saws) started shedding tears.

'Abdur-Rahman ibn 'Awf (ra) said: O Messenger of Allah, even you are weeping!

He said: O Ibn 'Awf, this is mercy.

Then he wept more and said: The eyes shed tears and the heart is grieved, and we will not say except what pleases our Lord. O Ibraheem! Indeed we are grieved by your separation." (Bukhari)

10   Bukhari and Muslim.

11   It was narrated from Jabir (ra) that the Messenger of Allah (saws) said:

"Whoever says: *Subhan Allahul-'Adheem wa bihamdihi* (glory and praise be to Allah, the Almighty), a palm tree will be planted for him in paradise." (at-Tirmidhi; graded *saheeh* by al-Albani)

12   Abu Moosa al-Ash'ari (ra) reported that the Messenger of Allah (saws) said:

"When the child of a servant dies, Allah asks the angels: Have you taken the life of My servant's child?

They say: Yes.

Allah asks: Have you taken the fruit of his heart?

They say: Yes.

Allah says: What has My servant said?

They say: He has praised You and said: to Allah we belong and to Allah we return.

Allah says: Build a house for My servant in paradise and name it the House of Praise." (at-Tirmidhi; graded *hasan* by al-Albani)

13   Bukhari.

14   'Adiy ibn Hatim (ra) heard the Prophet (saws) say:

"Save yourself from hellfire even by giving half a date in charity." (Bukhari)

15   It was narrated that 'Umar ibn al-Khattab (ra) said:

"Some prisoners were brought to the Messenger of Allah. Among them was a woman, searching. When she found a child among the prisoners, she took hold of it, pressed it against her chest, and nursed it.

The Messenger of Allah (saws) asked: Do you think this woman could ever manage to throw her child into the fire?

We said: By Allah, so far as it lies in her power, she would never throw her child into the fire!

The Messenger of Allah (saws) said: Allah has more compassion for His servants than this woman does for her child." (Muslim)

16   {Whatever you have will end, but what Allah has is lasting. And We will surely give those who were patient their reward according to the best of what they used to do.}   *(an-Naḥl 16:96)*

17   Abu Dawood; graded *saheeh* by al-Albani.

18   Ahmad; graded *saheeh* by al-Albani.

19   Abu Hurayrah (ra) reported that the Messenger of Allah (saws) said:

"Allah (swt) said: Whosoever shows enmity to someone devoted to Me, I shall be at war with him. My servant draws not near to Me with anything more loved by Me than the religious duties I have enjoined upon him, and My servant continues to draw near to Me with supererogatory works so that I shall love him.

When I love him I am his hearing with which he hears, his seeing with which he sees, his hand with which he grips and his foot with which he walks. Were he to ask (something) of Me, I would surely give it to him, and were he to ask Me for refuge, I would surely grant him it. I do not hesitate about anything as much as I hesitate about (seizing) the soul of My faithful servant: he hates death and I hate hurting him." (Bukhari)

20   It was narrated from Abu Salam (ra), the servant of the Prophet (saws), that the Prophet (saws) said:

"There is no Muslim – or no person, or slave (of Allah) – who says, in the morning and evening:

I am content with Allah as my Lord, with Islam as my religion, and with Muhammad as my prophet,

but he will have a promise from Allah to make him pleased on the Day of Resurrection." (Ahmad, at-Tirmidhi, and an-Nasa'i; graded *hasan* by Ibn Baz)

21   Abu Hurayrah (ra) reported that the Prophet (saws) said:

"There are seven people whom Allah will shade on a day when there is no shade but His. They are:
a just ruler,
a young person who grew up in the worship of Allah,
a person whose heart is attached to the mosques,
two persons who love each other who meet and depart from each other for the sake of Allah,
a man whom a beautiful woman of high status seduces but he rejects her by saying: I fear Allah,
a person who spends in charity and conceals it such that his right hand does not know what his left hand has given,
and a person who remembered Allah in private and he wept." (Bukhari and Muslim)

22   {Indeed, Allah [alone] has knowledge of the Hour and sends down the rain and knows what is in the wombs. And no soul perceives what it will earn tomorrow, and no soul perceives in what land it will die. Indeed, Allah is knowing and acquainted.}   *(Luqmân 31:34)*

23   at-Tirmidhi, who graded it hasan.

24   at-Tirmidhi; graded *saheeh* by al-Albani.

25 {And the day the wrongdoer will bite on his hands [in regret] he will say: Oh, I wish I had taken with the Messenger a way.} *(al-Furqân 25:27)*

26 Muslim.

27 Bukhari and Muslim.

28 Muslim.

29 at-Tirmidhi; graded *saheeh* by al-Albani.

30 Abu Hurayrah (ra) reported that the Messenger of Allah (saws) said:

"Whoever is wounded while fighting in the way of Allah will come on the Day of Resurrection with blood oozing from his wound having the colour of blood but with the fragrance of musk." (Bukhari and Muslim)

31 Abu Hurayrah (ra) reported that the Messenger of Allah (saws) said:

"Allah, the Exalted, said: Every deed of the son of Adam is for him except fasting, for it is done for My sake and I will reward it.

The Prophet (saws) added: By Allah, in whose hand is the soul of Muhammad, the breath of a fasting person is sweeter to Allah than the fragrance of musk." (Muslim)

32 Abu Hurayrah (ra) narrated that the Messenger of Allah (saws) said:

"The deeds (of humankind) are presented (to Allah) every Monday and Thursday, and I like my deeds to be presented (to Allah) while I am fasting." (at-Tirmidhi; graded *saheeh* by al-Albani)

33 It was narrated that Abu Dharr (ra) said:

"The Messenger of Allah (saws) said to me: If you fast any part of the month then fast on the thirteenth, fourteenth, and fifteenth." (al-Nasa'i; graded *saheeh* by al-Albani)

34 It was reported by 'Aishah (rah) that Prophet Muhammad (saws) said:

"The deeds most loved by Allah (swt) (are those) done regularly, even if they are small." (Bukhari and Muslim)

35 Muslim.

36 Bukhari.

37 "A man asked the Prophet (saws): When will the Hour be established, O Messenger of Allah?

The Prophet (saws) asked him: What have you prepared for it?

The man said: I haven't prepared for it much of prayers or fast or alms, but I love Allah and His Messenger.

The Prophet (saws) said: You will be with those whom you love." (Bukhari)

38   at-Tirmidhi, who graded it *hasan ghareeb*.

39   Qaroon was a wealthy and arrogant man from Moosa's people who rejected Allah's message. Allah caused the earth to swallow him.

40   Muslim.

41   The Messenger of Allah (saws) said:

"Three supplications will not be rejected: the supplication of the parent for his child, the supplication of the one who is fasting, and the supplication of the traveler." (Bayhaqi; graded *saheeh* by al-Albani)

42   Ibn Taymiyah (1263–1328 CE) was a renowned Islamic scholar and theologian, often referred to as the "Sheikh of Islam."

43   {Indeed, in the creation of the heavens and the earth and the alternation of the night and the day are signs for those of understanding.

Who remember Allah while standing or sitting or [lying] on their sides and give thought to the creation of the heavens and the earth, [saying]: Our Lord, You did not create this aimlessly; exalted are You [above such a thing]; then protect us from the punishment of the fire.}

(Âl-'Imrân 3:190-191)

44 Bukhari.

45 Muslim.

46 The People of the Cave were a group of young men who were persecuted for their monotheistic belief. They fled to a cave, where they fell asleep. According to the Qur'an, they slept for 309 years. When they awoke they discovered that the people of the city they had fled had become believers.
(al-Kahf 18: 9-26)

47 al-Bukhari.

48   Muslim.

49 {If We had sent down this Qur'an upon a mountain, you would have seen it humbled and coming apart from fear of Allah. And these examples We present to the people that perhaps they will give thought.}   *(al-Ḥashr 59:21)*

50 Bukhari.

51 Bukhari.

52   al-Hakim; graded *hasan saheeh* by al-Albani. At the hands of her tormentors, Sumayyah was the first martyr in Islam.

53   Sufyan ath-Thawri (716–778 CE) was a well-known scholar and compiler of hadith.

54   The Messenger of Allah (saws) said:

"Whenever a Muslim supplicates to Allah, He accepts his supplication or averts any similar kind of trouble from him until he prays for something sinful or something that may break the ties of kinship.

One of the Companions said: Then we shall supplicate plenty.

The Messenger of Allah (saws) said: Allah is more plentiful (in responding)." (at-Tirmidhi; graded *saheeh* by al-Albani)

55   Abu Hurayrah (ra) reported that the Prophet (saws) said:

"Hardships continue to befall a believing man and woman in their body, family, and property, until they meet Allah burdened with no sins." (at-Tirmidhi; graded *saheeh* by al-Albani)

56   Sulayman ibn Qasim was an Egyptian zahid, or ascetic. Quoted in Ibn Abi ad-Dunya, *as-Sabr wath-Thawab 'Alayhi,* 29.

57   {O you who have believed, seek help through patience and prayer. Indeed, Allah is with the patient.}   *(al-Baqarah 2:153)*

58   {Say: O My servants who have believed, fear your Lord. For those who do good in this world is good, and the earth of Allah is spacious. Indeed, the patient will be given their reward without account.}   *(az-Zumar 39:10)*

59   Muslim.

60   {Except for those who repent, believe, and do righteous work. For them Allah will replace their evil deeds with good. And ever is Allah forgiving and merciful.}   *(al-Furqân 25:70)*

61   Bukhari and Muslim.

62   Bukhari and Muslim.

63   {Have you not considered that Allah knows what is in the heavens and what is on the earth? There is in no private conversation three but that He is the fourth of them, nor are there five but that He is the sixth of them – and no less than that and no more except that He is with them [in knowledge] wherever they are. Then He will inform them of what they did, on the Day of Resurrection. Indeed Allah is, of all things, knowing.}

(al-Mujâdilah 58:7)

64   Muslim.

65   Ibn Mas'ood (ra) reported that the Messenger of Allah (saws) said:

"I met Ibraheem (as) on the Night of Ascension and he said to me: O Muhammad! Convey my greetings to your nation, and tell them that paradise has a vast plain of pure soil and sweet water and is set as a plain leveled land. The plants grow there by [a believer] uttering: *Subhan Allah, wa alhamdu lillah, wa la ilaha ill-Allah, wa Allahu akbar.*" (at-Tirmidhi, who graded it *hasan*)

66   *Ibrâheem 14:41* and *al-Isrâ' 17:24.*

About the Author

Asmaa Hussein is a writer, registered social worker, and mother of a spirited daughter. Her children's titles include "Bismillah Soup" and "Yasmine's Belly Button." She is also the creator of Ruqaya's Bookshelf, a website about Islamic parenting. Asmaa has a BA in English and Sociology and a MA in Social Work. She was born and raised in Toronto, Canada and has been actively involved in the Muslim community there for many years. She currently lives in Toronto with her family.